Seen, Heard & Understood

Parenting & Partnering with Teens for Greater Mental Health

Seen, Heard & Understood

Parenting & Partnering with Teens for Greater Mental Health

By

Lainie Liberti

Foreword by Miro Siegel

Praise For:

Seen, Heard & Understood

"Lainie Liberti provides relief from the fear-based need to control your teen, allowing partnership to replace domination. With a validating voice, she provides tools to heal yourself, such that you don't have to react to your teen from your pain, but respond from your love."

~**Naomi Aldort,** Author of Raising Our Children, Raising Ourselves; Transforming Parent-Child Relationship from Reaction and Struggle to Freedom, Power and Joy

"Do you feel there must be a better way to live with your teenager, but don't know how to start? This book could be just what you need. A powerful call to parents to look directly at young people, listen to where they are coming from and support them to find the life they want to lead. Combining personal experience, neuroscientific research and practical tools, Lainie guides you towards a different way of being with your teen, moving from coercion and manipulation to partnership and connection."

~**Dr. Naomi Fisher,** Clinical Psychologist and Author of Changing Our Minds: How Children Can Take Control of their Own Learning

"What Lainie Liberti and her son, Miro have accomplished as a mom and son team, especially with Project World School, is fantastic, amazing, and awe-inspiring! What made their adventure of a lifetime possible was parent-child connection built on a growing and deepening secure parent-child attachment relationship. Lainie refers to this as partnership or facilitator parenting, something that doesn't come easy for parents who grew up in authoritarian systems. Lainie had to courageously face and challenge the triggers of her own childhood trauma in order to make that deep connection with her son. Lainie 's book reassures parents that you and your child CAN build this connection, too! She gently challenges parents to explore the childhood traumas in their own pasts that lead them to become triggered by their wonderful adolescents today. Lainie's book is packed with tools and worksheets to help parents and adolescents improve their relationship,

understand one another, deepen their connection, and expand the bounds of freedom for both... Imagine what wonderful adventures you and your child can discover or even invent as a result!"

    ~Laurie A. Couture, Author of Instead of Medicating and Punishing: Healing the Causes of Our Children's Acting-Out Behavior By Parenting and Educating the Way Nature Intended and the upcoming book, Nurturing and Empowering Our Sons.

"What's Lainie's magic formula? Mixing her reflections on her own hard experiences combined with an extensive study of developmental psychology. Her presentation led me to reflect on my own upbringing, my parenting choices, and my professional work with teens over the past three decades. Lainie's thoughtful synthesis and useful set of tools will support each of us in making a difference for families."

    ~Kenneth Danford, Executive Director, North Star: Self-Directed Learning for Teens

"Finally.. a book that sees and understands the unique needs of teenagers without all the negative stereotypes. This book is a gem."

    ~Christiane Northrup, M.D., New York Times best-selling author of Goddesses Never Age, The Wisdom of Menopause, and Women's Bodies, Women's Wisdom

"As a mom of two teenagers, and a longtime admirer of Lainie Liberti's work, I value her insights on prioritizing connection over coercion in our parenting approach. Seen, Heard & Understood provides the tools and inspiration to build a powerful, peaceful partnership with our teens."

    ~Kerry McDonald, Author of Unschooled: Raising Curious, Well-Educated Children Outside the Conventional Classroom

"This book is a major contribution to unschooling and homeschooling families and to the movement for reimagining education. It names the proverbial elephant in the room. Unless we as parents heal our own

intergenerational trauma and face our fears and anxieties, we risk passing these to our children. Born out of many years of hands-on experience, this book offers very practical tools for how we can enter into partnership parenting and build a genuine learning culture with our teens centered around freedom and accountability. It is a powerful post-Covid roadmap for navigating the inner world of our teens and ourselves as adults. Lainie Liberti has gifted us with the parent's liberation handbook for our times.

~**Manish Jain,** Co-Founder of the Swaraj University, Learning Societies Network and Shikshantar: The Peoples' Institute for Rethinking Education and Development of Udaipur, India

"Lainie's book is such a vital read and all the more so at this current moment in time. Studies are coming in from around the world highlighting unprecedented numbers of young people who are struggling with depression, anxiety, and other mental and physical illnesses. Many teens are worn down by society at such an early age but we can change this by listening to the ideas in this book. Having parents or caregivers who understand their needs and developmental stages and who can help encourage and support in such caring ways as Lainie outlines, can be life changing (or life-saving). This book provides the research and theoretical background in understandable and applied ways and is like a warm, snuggly blanket for parents who want to help their youth but feel overwhelmed. The processes and works outlined lead to such in depth change for the entire family system. I fully recommend digging into this for anyone who is a parent or works with young people."

~**Dr. Kate Green**, PhD Developmental Psychology

"There is no one who knows teenagers better than Lainie Liberti. She cares deeply about them and wants them to always feel seen, heard, and understood. If you are a parent, a guardian, or an individual who works with adolescents, this book is a must read. It is one of the most kind, gentle, and wise books on teens and teen behavior that I have ever read."

~**Gina Riley,** Ph.D. Clinical Professor of Adolescent Special Education

City University of New York - Hunter College and author of
Unschooling: Exploring Learning Beyond the Classroom

"When it comes right down to it, we all just want to be seen, heard and understood so we can lead our lives in the most authentic way possible. This book is positively bursting with scientific research, practical information, personal guidance, and heartfelt advice for any parents raising the mysterious and beautiful beings known as teens. Reading this book will not only change your relationship with your teen but challenge your assumptions about yourself as a parent in the most positive and beneficial of ways."

~**Jeremy Stuart,** Filmmaker, Class Dismissed: A Film About Learning Outside of the Classroom and Self-Taught: Life Stories From Self-Directed Learners

"What a thought-provoking, enjoyable and easy read this book is! Lainie Liberti presents to her readers a transformative guide on how to be in partnership with your teens. Especially as you navigate building your relationship with them based on trust, understanding and deep knowledge of each other. If you have pre-teens/teens in your life, this book is a must read!"

~**Erika Davis-Pitre,** President, HSC-Homeschool Association of California

"I'm so happy Lainie has written this fabulous book! She shares so many tools to help parents of teens navigate through adolescence. I've known Lainie for years - always connecting with teens, seeing them, listening to them and really understanding them! And now, through this book, so many more will benefit from her wisdom, passion, and insight!"

~**Sue Patterson,** Parenting Coach & Author of Homeschooled Teens: 75 Young People Speak about their Lives without School

"Seen, Heard & Understood is an exciting must-read for parents interested in supporting their teens through partnership for greater mental health. This book offers practical, insightful strategies and exercises for families interested in a non-authoritarian approach to parenting. I highly recommend it for parents rethinking their current paradigm, for adolescents looking for a better way to relate to their parents, and for potential future parents who seek to nurture the next generation of well rounded young adults. With this book, parents and adolescents can heal the wounds from their childhood and reshape the trajectory of the world."

~Derrick Broze, Journalist, Founder of The Conscious Resistance Network

"Humanity is in the midst of a tidal wave of change. Old paradigms are crumbling. A more beautiful new world is emerging. In the area of education and parenting, many conscious families are stepping into a more respectful partnership-based paradigm. We're letting go of old ways based on control and behavior modification, and choosing the new paradigm based on kindness, respect, and mutual understanding. In doing so, we're healing on all levels and creating a more peaceful world where humanity can blossom into our fullest possibilities.

For parents who resonate with this new paradigm, Lainie's book is an absolute treasure trove of gifts! Weaving together inspirational stories with science-backed tools, Lainie takes you on a rich and insightful journey, so that you can navigate your own parenting path with greater courage, wisdom, and inner clarity. Highly recommended for parents of teens who value sovereignty, respect, and freedom. Highly recommended for all families who wish to cocreate a more kind, compassionate, and peaceful world."

~Dr. Edith Ubuntu Chan, Consciousness & Human Potential coach, Author of "SuperWellness" & upcoming book "Luminous Kids"

For Miro, who inspired me to be the best version of myself. You gave me a reason to get down and dirty, look at my shit, and really, really heal. You are the best reason this book exists and I do the work I do. I love you to the moon and back.

...and for teenage Lainie, who lives within.
You are now finally seen, heard, and understood.

Contents

Foreword
By Miro Siegel

Like many other parents, my mother had to learn the contents of this book for herself over the course of my childhood. It was (and still is) a process of trial and error, during which many mistakes were made and many lessons learned. At times this was incredibly difficult and sometimes messy, because my mom is not a perfect parent nor is she a perfect being. No, instead she was something far greater; she was always human.

Growing up, I never had the near mythological idea of my parents that so many of my friends had of theirs. My friends had parents who could do no wrong, whose say was final, who demanded respect unconditionally. My friends had parents who in their relationships more closely resembled gods than they did people, and how does one learn accountability and vulnerability from a god? My experience couldn't have been any more different; instead of an iron fist, I was raised with tenderness and transparency in a partnership paradigm.

In my family, I was able to practice valuable skills like negotiation and compromise, something that was only possible because my mom was ok with being wrong from time to time. I realized that no one was entitled to my respect or trust, because my mom never demanded it, but earned it instead. Through my mom I learned that it was okay to be wrong, to apologize and to admit my own shortcomings in order to grow. Through watching her, I learned how to improve myself and how to genuinely connect with others. Instead of hindering me, our family dynamic prepared me for the relationships I would have later on in my life.

The beauty of having an authentic parent is that it prepares us for the inevitability of our own imperfections and allows us to see others for who they are, not who we want them to be.

As I've grown into my early adulthood, I have been faced with near constant reminders of my own imperfections. This is not a complaint, but simply an unspoken and natural part of life that everyone experiences at some point. Instead of being set back by these reminders, I am fueled by them. I think of my mother, her beautiful flaws and the way she worked on herself throughout my childhood. She modeled self-love and patience openly, and I witnessed it every day. She never needed to fix me, fixing herself was more than enough.

And while my mom was always there for me first, her compassion could not be contained and was not limited to her own son. I can't even begin to recount all of her selfless acts of kindness over the years. She connected with teens and listened to them when they felt they had no one else and she answered emails (likely in the thousands) from families who needed guidance. She changed the trajectory of people's lives, people she had never even met or previously interacted with, without ever expecting anything in return.

This book (like every other project my mom develops for teens) is a true labor of love, written as much for others as it was for herself. In this book, everything I mentioned above is on full display: her vulnerability, her strength of character and her genuine interest and passion for teens. Alongside the extensive research, philosophy and information contained in these pages, my mom has also fully given herself to you, the reader.

I am a living testimony to the contents of this book, and I couldn't be any happier with who I've become. They say being a mother is a thankless job, but that doesn't feel right here. Thank you, mom.

Chapter 1: Introduction

No one ever said adolescence was easy.

It is not an easy stage for a young person to pass through, nor is it easy on the parent. But it can be rewarding for both the parents and teens if connection is the priority. Recognizing the ups and downs, the struggles and triumphs, as well as the perceptions and tendencies of this stage will help us as parents to remain connected and supportive.

Parents, I am writing this book for you. I am writing this book from one parent to another, to affect as much positive change in the world as possible, starting first with you and your family. I am writing this book so you will have the tools to support your teens with confidence in a rapidly changing world. I am writing this book so you will have the tools to become a supportive partner in your teens' lives. The intention of this book is to help you recognize how your internal reactions, beliefs, and expectations affect the relationship you wish to create with your teen and to provide tools to help you become accountable to your teen and to yourself.

This book is written during the time of the COVID-19 pandemic when the world around us looks very different than it did pre-2020. It is important to note that as a result of lockdowns, restrictions, social divisiveness, education disruptions, and radical changes within every area of our society, adolescents around the world have felt the repercussions in countless and unforeseen ways. Numerous psychological studies are starting to reveal that due to the social effects of the pandemic, there has been an exponential increase in adolescent suicide, anxiety, depression, and various other consequences. The timing of this book couldn't be more welcome, and even if your teen is not experiencing psychological disruptions, they are living in a world where this reality is ever increasing.

There was no book like this available for me when I started to parent an adolescent. I was terrified to make the same mistakes my parents did and wasn't sure how to handle the big changes we know as the teenage years. My hope is to connect with other parents, so they know they are not alone on their journey, and they are supported by someone who took the path of self-healing and cares deeply about empowering youth through this stage of their life. I wrote this book to help you build your confidence in knowing you can do this too.

I want to share with you the insights I've learned from working with hundreds of teens and help you to conceptualize what the partnership journey can look like. I wrote this book to develop a culture of greater emotional intelligence and to help heal families' generational wounds. I wrote this book because it is especially needed in the world right now.

I recognize how trite it sounds when someone says, "If I can do it, you can do it." But you can because you've got skin in the game. If the sanity and mental health of your teen is at stake, then you need to show up for them in a way they can relate to. I wrote this book so you can do just that. I'm going to say it…

"You can do this!"

It is just as important to be clear about what this book won't do. This book will **not** teach you how to modify your teen's behavior to better suit your comfort or desires. This book will **not** teach you how to manipulate your teen into being more of *something* or less of *something else* just because it's what you think is best for them. On the flip side, this book will challenge you to be accountable for your own agendas and help you to release those expectations, empowering you to see your teen for who they actually are in this very moment, rather than who you think they should be or once were.

I was born into what I thought was a typical American family. At the time, I thought my childhood was normal and everyone experienced the world as I did. Growing up, I had not been granted the gift of kindness, tenderness, or connection and thought everyone's journey looked the same as mine. Later,

I was shocked to realize my childhood was filled with countless traumas, attachment wounds, emotional neglect, and abuse.

Of course, the effects played out through my adolescence and well into my adulthood. My predominant experience throughout my teen years was that I was invisible and I didn't matter to my family, myself, or the world. Never once in my teen years did I feel seen, heard, or understood by any family member or any adult in my life.

Years of unpacking, self-inquiry, healing, and integrating these core wounds propelled me into a journey deep into myself. I recognized the most self-destructive period of my journey was my own adolescence. I often reflect on how different my life could have been had I been supported, had tools to process my emotions and challenge my beliefs about myself, or had I simply been "seen."

I wrote this book to help more teens be seen, heard, and understood. I wrote this book to help their parents who love them to have the tools to do this with ease and grace. What qualifies me to write a book of this nature?

I don't have a formal degree in psychology, parenting, childhood development, or therapy. However, I was born with the insatiable desire to learn and have always dived deep into the topics I was interested in.

In my childhood, I discovered the wealth of knowledge in libraries, where I spent a great portion of my time. I was exposed to a world of imagination, where I discovered and loved everything about creativity and art. During my early years, I immersed myself in modern art and art history. I explored many contemporary art movements like surrealism, dadaism, conceptual, and performance art, and the modern art movement. I studied in the library and explored the local art museums and regional galleries. I started making art myself, and by the time I enrolled in college to study art, I already had the equivalent of an art history degree based on the feedback and conversations I had with my professors.

Later, I changed career paths and started working as a graphic designer in commercial advertising and marketing. However, the discipline of branding caught my interest after a few years. I studied the principles, concepts, theories, and practices of branding. I read every book and case study I could get my hands on. Although I had no official training in the field, I was knowledgeable enough after a few years to open my own successful branding agency in Los Angeles, which I owned, operated, and directed for over eight years.

During my late twenties and early thirties, I started to recognize many significant patterns showing up in my interpersonal relationships. My fierce independence was something I always considered to be one of my superpowers, but I soon recognized it was masking my fear of intimacy and the limiting beliefs I had about myself. Then, at thirty-two, I found myself pregnant. I knew the greatest gift I could give my unborn son was to uncover and heal some of my early traumas and learn how to be the parent to him I never had.

I always felt empowered to learn things through research and identified as an autodidact. This gave me the confidence to set out on a journey to heal while learning everything I could absorb about psychology, trauma, neuroscience and brain biology, parenting, and self-healing techniques. So that's what I did. I learned through acquiring knowledge, and I learned through experience. Over the next twenty years, my priority had become to learn, to go deeper, to explore, and heal myself, my relationships, and my soul. This book is a testament to that journey. You will find many of the resources I used along the way at the end of this book.

For those who have been following me over the years, this part of my story will be of no surprise, but it's important to include in this book's intro for those who don't know me.

By 2008, I had been running my own branding agency for eight years. My client list had grown as I developed a wonderful reputation for uniquely serving green-eco companies and a handful of well-known nonprofits. But as 2008 came to a close, the California economy was in collapse, and I saw the majority of my clients drop away one by one. I knew change was coming, but I didn't know exactly what.

From the time my son was born, I have been a single parent. My son's father was in his life until he passed away, but he struggled with health issues and was not often available as a result. I was the custodial parent and responsible for my son Miro's everything: education, health decisions, and emotional and social well-being.

As you can imagine, I worked a lot. In fact, as a business owner and the agency's creative director, I worked upwards of 60 hours per week. One of the most common phrases I heard come out of my son's mouth was, "Mom, you are always working. You never spend any time with me." As a parent, my heart broke into a million tiny pieces every time he spoke those words.

One night, late in 2008, nine-year-old Miro and I were sitting in the office. I was feeling stressed, overworked, and completely burned out. Knowing I wasn't going to bring my staff back in 2009, I looked over at Miro, who was playing video games on one of the office computers. I turned to him and said, "Miro, let's get rid of all our stuff. Let's go have an adventure!" He looked up from his games and said, "Ok! Let's do it!"

And that was that. It took us six months to sell or give away most of our possessions. Then we shoved the remainder of our belongings into two very heavy backpacks and set out for what was meant to be one year of travel.

As usual, I researched, learned, and prepared. I read books like *The 4-Hour Workweek*, *Vagabonding*, and *The Power of Now.* I studied guides for Central and South America and off we went.

That one-year trip turned into thirteen years (and counting).

Throughout our years of travel, we adapted "unschooling" or "self-directed learning" as our form of education. As a parent, I took my role in the process seriously, further adapting a partnership paradigm in learning and life, being the best facilitator for my son, listening to his cues, offering support, providing resources, and committing to learning right alongside him. We were conscious of this choice and took on the task of learning intentionally.

From the start of our journey, we made joint decisions about our lives, deciding where to go, when to go, and how to live. We opted for living in true partnership, and both of our needs were being met as we learned to collaborate and adjust along the way.

Years later, we spearheaded the growing "worldschooling" movement through our advocacy and community organization.

Over the years, Miro and I slow-traveled through dozens of countries. We lived like visiting locals, deeply immersing ourselves in the cultures we lived in, volunteering, exploring, and living life together. We even spoke about our lives on the TEDx Edu stage in Amsterdam in 2016 in front of a live audience of 400 people. We spoke about our unique way of being in the world and learning through travel.

We practiced partnership as the key to our family culture and approached learning as a fluid experience we were both responsible for. We became equal partners in all decisions including travel, budgeting, and life. We even launched a company together called Project World School.

Project World School was born in 2012. The idea was to create inspiring temporary learning communities around the world for teens, by providing a safe space to be in a community, have an adventure, and learn from the world. I designed a program, a way of being in a community focused on extending secure attachment principles to the adolescent experience. Project World School retreats empower teens to step out of their comfort zones in safety (risk-taking), question everything (rebellion), work in collaboration (social learning), and strive for consensus within a community setting.

Once again, I studied, read, listened, and learned everything I could; this time focusing on community building, facilitation, team building, social learning, and conflict resolution. I also expanded my knowledge about psychology and adolescent development, learning more about the teen brain. This body of information was distilled into a program combining experiential learning in a space where teens were seen, heard, and understood. Early on, I recognized that facilitating teens in community is a nuanced challenge and realized that the healing tools I learned and practiced in my own life would certainly come in handy.

For the first several years of Project World School, Miro participated as one of the teens and thrived within a community of his peers, something he craved deeply. Over the years, Miro stepped into greater roles of responsibility within the retreats as he became more comfortable co-facilitating with me.

Since 2012, we have facilitated more than twenty international retreats in countries like Thailand, Greece, Wales, Peru, Japan, Mexico, and South Africa for almost one-hundred teens. Living and working in community with teens has been tremendously healing for me, as I've been able to create the very thing I did not have growing up, a safe space to be a teen. These experiences have empowered me to recognize the challenges of adolescence and have given me the opportunity to connect with teens in spaces where they needed connection. This is the space and the spirit in which I write this book for you.

I am not a doctor. There are no strings of letters behind my name. I am writing this book as a self-educated, passionate student of this topic. I have spent countless hours diving into the nature of the adolescent brain through my novice lens and have spent as many hours distilling the information I've absorbed into practical applications and tools to help myself and others demystify and befriend the inner workings of oneself.

I was born a little over 50 years ago, raised by hippies who were born into the Boomer generation. This generation came of age in the 60s and 70s and was oftentimes referred to as the "me generation."

The "me generation" often ascribed higher importance to exploring and achieving self-realization over social responsibility, or in my case, family responsibility. I was raised by an absent father, who was out of the house most days working to support his family, and a young mother, whose highest pursuit and priority was to find herself.

Being born to parents of the "me generation" certainly impacted my emotional development and likely affected an entire generation. Latchkey kids were on the rise, and my generation was the first to be raised through television programming and with less human connection than the generations before.

My mother was introduced to yoga in the 1970s, and she studied with vigor, eventually becoming a yoga teacher. Throughout my childhood, I was dragged to her gurus' talks, ashrams, and classes, and even dragged off to spend time with her yoga friends, some of whom she was romantically involved with.

Although I don't believe my mother was formally diagnosed as being a narcissist, upon reflection, I experienced her as such. Many things pointed to this, and it wasn't until adulthood that I made that connection. For example, my mother had commissioned a portrait artist to paint an eight-foot oil painting of herself posing nude, kneeling, as if she was an omnipotent ruler. This painting hung prominently in her bedroom, and throughout my childhood, I saw her as a kneeling god I was born to please. But she never found any joy in my presence. My mother-god's needs, wishes, and desires were always the most dominant priority in our family, and my or my brother's interests were never considered.

Even though my mother's pursuit to find herself was her priority, she still had a highly controlling approach to her home. There were protocols for behavior, daily chores, and distinct rules about cleaning. There were punishments associated with doing chores incorrectly. Most rules were arbitrary, like learning the differences between 'garbage' and 'trash.' I assumed everyone knew that garbage was ALWAYS to be thrown outside in the garbage can on the side of the house. On the other hand, trash could be left in the house, until the waste-paper baskets were emptied. If I was caught putting 'garbage' into the trash can, I could expect (and received on multiple occasions) the entire contents of the trash to be emptied out on my bedroom floor. Then, I was made to clean it up.

I was yelled at almost on a daily basis, as I always did something wrong. I recall the feeling of my tiny body shaking in proximity to her violent screams. Throughout my childhood and into my adolescence, I often slept with all my blankets completely covering my head. This was my bastion of security and one of the only safe spaces I felt I could cry.

As an adult, I cannot recall any tender moments with my mother, nor do I remember any acts of kindness from her as a child. For many years, I simply thought all of this was normal.

Although this is only one of the volumes of the formative experiences I had, I wanted to give you an idea of the type of wounds I had to overcome. Learning to face these wounds and heal them has been one of my greatest gifts. Learning how my early childhood experiences informed the adolescent and the adult I grew into provided me with much insight into the healing of the human psyche.

"An environment that is not safe to disagree in is not an environment focused on growth- it's an environment focused on control."

~ Wendi Jade

Since the beginning of 2020, I've heard from parents of teens and tweens around the world that this pandemic has served up challenges and changes that they (and their teens) were just not equipped to handle.

Many of the teens I've been working with have shared their frustrations too, that the only choice they have is to just move through it. Many have shared the feelings of just shutting down, not really caring about the things they used to be passionate about, as a way to handle the deeper sense of loss. These feelings oftentimes are internalized without any natural outlet, leaving them bubbling just beneath the surface.

I get it. I really do. It's so difficult in a time when teens should be expressing their independence.

Many parents see this emotion below the surface become expressed through their teen's behavior, which can look like anger, withdrawal, rebellion, depression, self-sabotage, self-harm, or anxiety. Justifiably so, most parents must navigate a new way of being in the world too, often with financial and logistic implications and tend to react to what's directly in front of them: their teen's behavior.

What will you find in this book?

This book aims to provide a basic understanding of two main things. First, is the nature of adolescent development including brain, emotional, psychological, and mental changes. The second is a basic idea of how to support and facilitate teens by using the powerful tools provided in the last half of this book.

This book is written specifically for you, the parent of adolescents, and I will especially be addressing your part of the equation. But be warned, for some, the material in this book will trigger your unresolved childhood wounds as you uncover limiting beliefs developed in your own youth. With that said, please approach this journey as a path to your own healing. There is a robust reference section at the end of this book, so if you wish to go deeper into your own personal development journey, you will have the necessary support and resources to start that process.

Also, throughout this book, I will share many stories from my own childhood, adolescence, self-directed learning, and my healing journey. Wherever you are starting from, let's begin from there. Your teen is counting on you!

How do you use this book?

The tools in this book will not only allow you to facilitate your teen's mental health journey but also take time to check in first and be accountable for your own mental health. For example, it is impossible to facilitate emotional intelligence without developing your own emotional intelligence. It's difficult to facilitate a teen through questioning and reprogramming their own limiting beliefs without first doing it yourself. I invite you to use this book as a reference to be the healthiest version of you as possible, in order for you to have the insight to facilitate the mental health journey with your teen. My recommendation for you is to first read through this book, dog-ear, bookmark, highlight passages, do the exercises, use the tools, and journal your experiences.

Note on the use of the terms "adolescence" and "teens" throughout this book:

Adolescence is the stage of development in a person's life, ranging roughly from ages 10 to 25, in which physical and psychological development takes place from the onset of puberty to adulthood.

Throughout this book, I use the term "adolescent" at times, and at others, I use the terms "teen" or "teenager," in order to make the words more readable and relatable. I understand the term "teen" or "teenager" is not accurate in terms of denoting a numeric age, but I ask you to recognize these words are referencing the median age of adolescence and do not exclude ages 10-12 or 20-25.

Adolescence is a pivotal time in a person's development, and many psychologists specialize in this stage. Because adolescence is a time of rapidly changing emotional states, sexual maturation, puberty, physical growth, and social changes, researchers in this area specialize in issues unique to adolescents like gender, sexual development, and cognitive and behavioral development. For a list of resources, please check the Suggested Reading section for more reading recommendations.

Chapter 2: A Seen, Heard & Understood Mindset

Adapting a seen, heard, and understood mindset is your mission throughout this book, and you can incorporate these tools into your family culture. But I must warn you, it takes a lot of work and self-awareness to cultivate in your own mind and translate it into your conscious interactions with your teens. Practice asking yourself, "Do my words and actions with my teen communicate that they are seen, heard, and understood?" Or could it be perceived as a judgment, control, or dismissal? Notice I said "perceived"? You are not ultimately responsible for how others interpret your words or actions, but you are responsible to learn how to interact in a way that promotes connection. I admit, it's a delicate dance we must take on as parents, and we don't always get it right, but there's connective power in making another person feel seen, heard, and understood.

However, in normal times, when the world around us is perceived as stable, making our teens feel seen, heard, and understood is nothing less than the greatest challenge.

Before we can go deeper in this book, we need to look at the collective trauma of living in a time of uncertainty. Let's face it, there has never been a time in most of our lives quite like what the pandemic has brought, and there's a lot going on. I've had many conversations with teens, parents, friends, and peers about the uncertainty we're all feeling, and no one is exempt from the psychological toll it continues to take.

Now that we are faced with so many uncertainties as a result of the global pandemic, changes we could have never anticipated pre-2020, we need to consider that you, I, your teens, and everyone we know is experiencing a collective trauma we could have never prepared for. I wanted to start this chapter by providing you with a simple tool to help you understand the nature of trauma and its stages as a framework to help you unpack and process the experiences we are having.

31

When I present this topic in my teen courses, one of my teens suggested I call this the "Trauma Train."

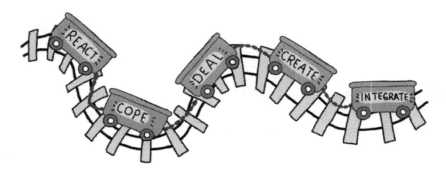

TRAUMA TRAIN

Where are you on the trauma train?

The Trauma Train has five distinguishable stages.

Stage One: React

During the first stage, we experience heightened sensations from an array of emotions, which command action or reaction. For example, many reacted or responded to the first news of the pandemic by agreeing to quarantine at home, to "flatten the curve." Another reaction we saw was many people purchased an excess amount of toilet paper. The response to a situation driven by heightened emotions (in the case above might be defined as fear) gives a sense of having some control we subconsciously perceive as not having any control over.

Stage Two: Cope

During the second stage, we find ways to cope. Some of us became overachievers, worked hard, took the opportunity to catch up on projects, and took up new hobbies. I remember reading so many posts during the early pandemic of countless people taking up making sourdough, focusing on new gardening projects, and some of us even started new businesses. There are just as many people who approach coping by checking out, binge-watching shows, or playing video games. All are methods of coping with the new isolation and changes in the world and are really similar in the sense that they provide a sense of control over the situation, similar to stage one.

Stage Three: Deal

The third stage on the Trauma Train is accepting that things have changed. It's an overwhelming feeling of grief and loss. Processing change often initiates us to ask, "Now what?" prompting us to search the depths of our being. This stage is usually experienced internally, and if the person experiencing it is not comfortable facing their emotions, it could look like numbing out. Many can feel depression and despair and may get stuck in this stage if there is no support system to process the emotions and accompanying thoughts.

Stage Four: Create

Stage four is the space where we get on with things and consciously decide to create something new. Unlike the coping stage where we may use starting a business as a tool to help us avoid feeling whatever we are feeling, the fourth stage is an actual retooling or refocusing of our point of reality. On the flip side, many don't feel empowered to believe something new is possible and spend very little time here, but others see this as a great opportunity to embody the phoenix rising from the ashes and begin anew.

Stage Five: Integrate

The last step of all trauma work is integration. However, it is virtually impossible to integrate trauma, make sense of our experiences, and combine the lessons into who we are and how we make sense of the world while we are still in trauma. This stage will be left as our work in the future, and my sincere hope is we create some systems through which we can all process trauma collectively.

The Trauma Train is not a linear experience. In fact, sometimes the Trauma Train feels like a rollercoaster. Oftentimes, we find ourselves propelled into the different stages out of sequence at a moment's notice. It's useful to have tools to process these experiences. This gives us a unique perspective as it relates to the COVID-19 pandemic. We are all experiencing it through different lenses of perception. For some of us, the restrictions in our location are more severe, and for others, they are not affecting us personally as much. However, the world we participate in has changed, and we are affected directly or indirectly.

Emotions

Emotions are one of the primary components of the Trauma Train, and I want to take a little time to break down the nature of emotions to help you support yourself and your teen, especially when big emotions emerge.

When you don't want to deal with those repressed emotions

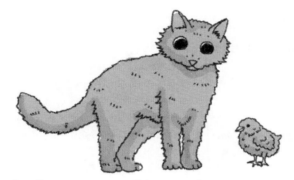

A few months later...

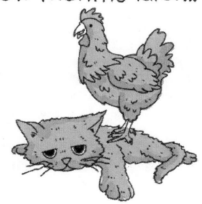

Unprocessed emotions are also referred to as repressed or unresolved emotions, and they can cause havoc on our mental health. Oftentimes, we push aside emotions we perceive as negative and overwhelming because we don't have the tools (or desire) to deal with them. A little later in this chapter, I will talk about the comfort zone and the stretch zone, and I've heard many teens describe their experience of facing negative emotions as outside of their comfort zone. That's really okay. Encourage your teen to get uncomfortable. The goal is to help you and your teen create a more positive relationship with their emotions.

1. **Emotions are natural.** Every human has the capacity to feel emotions. They are the biological function of our brains and serve a purpose. They come from within, and although they may feel painful or stressful at times, they are a natural part of the human experience.

2. **Emotions are temporary.** You are not always going to be in the emotional state you may be experiencing now, and different emotions come into your experience over a period of time. Just as they come in, they go away too. So, the desire to suppress emotions is not necessary because they're temporary in nature.

3. **Emotions are valid.** Giving yourself permission to see them as such changes the opposition to feeling them. It's not right; it's not wrong. You can allow yourself to feel it because you know it's natural and temporary. Everything else that comes up as a result of the emotion is valid and real. It's not made up. The fact that you're feeling it makes it real. So why argue with reality?

4. **Emotions provide information.** Because you are having an emotional response to something, you are learning about your perception. Maybe there is a misalignment with one of your core values or a limiting belief you haven't healed is triggered. Maybe you have sadness around the death of certain hopes and dreams, and it's an indication you must mourn. Emotions provide valuable information because they happen to us for a reason.

5. **Emotions are not facts.** There is no equal sign linking emotion to belief. For example, if you are feeling hurt, it doesn't prove you are unlovable. However, because emotions usually charge a thought or belief, emotions keep these thoughts or beliefs anchored in our minds. But they are just that, emotions temporarily visiting our body and they do not prove anything one way or another.

6. **Emotions are neither good nor bad.** How is that possible? It's totally natural to want to place a judgment or value on the thing you're feeling. But if we are feeling this thing, it's a natural thing. It's a temporary thing. It's valid; it's information; it's not based in fact. It's also not good or bad. If we shift our perception of what it feels like to be uncomfortable toward something that's exciting, it will no longer have a negative connotation. Then, we can just accept the feeling or the emotion for what it is, without judgment. Without this judgment or qualification, it is just a feeling visiting us temporarily.

7. **Emotions provide instruction.** They might be telling us it's time to do something or guiding us on what to do next. It is trying to give you the information needed to recognize it's time to change, act, or create, which we will discuss more in-depth in Chapter 6.

One of the tools I introduce to the teens I work with is this emotions wheel. It's a great representation of the grouping of emotions, and by getting specific with the exact emotion we are feeling, we develop greater emotional intelligence.

Here's a simple exercise to help develop greater emotional awareness:

1. My body is now feeling (emotion) _____.
2. My heart is now feeling (emotion) _____.
3. My mind is now feeling (emotion) _____.
4. My soul is now feeling (emotion) _____.
5. I am (emotion) _____.

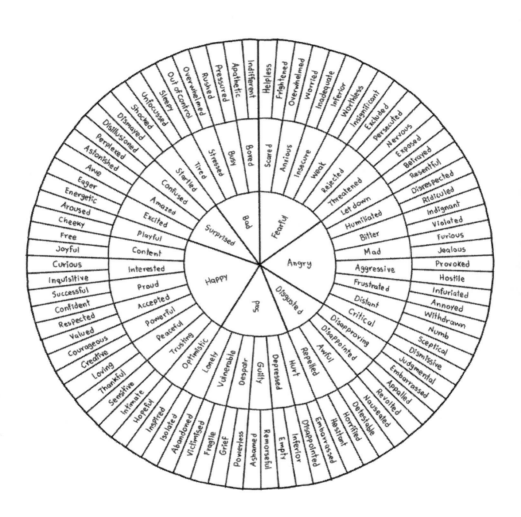

Supporting Our Teens on the Road to Adulthood

Now, more than ever, our teens need a supportive foundation from which to experience and know safety and security. Also, they desperately need tools to normalize greater awareness of their internal worlds by supporting a positive relationship with their own mental, emotional, and spiritual health, as well as their holistic well-being.

Your role in this process? That of the "facilitator."

The good news is you can enter into a partnership paradigm with your adolescent from this day forward, regardless of the current state of your relationship. However, it requires work from within you, the parent, and your willingness to step into your own journey. For some, that journey may be one of healing– it sure was for me. For many, this will also require a new approach to parenting that you'll learn about and explore throughout this book.

You will soon discover that in order to support your teens, you must commit to embarking on this journey together, with them by your side. This book is designed to hold you accountable within a partnership parenting paradigm, which will be explained more in the next section.

Partnering *with* your teen will help ease the stress of normal developmental changes, as well as help your family understand the challenges of growing up during a time of uncertainty. For many of us, the childhood we knew from an outer-world perspective was far more stable than our children have today. Many adolescents are trying to reconcile what it means to look towards a life that no longer meets their social expectations. Most are looking at a very different world with greater restrictions, fewer in-person social opportunities, and the reduction of the rites of passage we all came to expect like dances, travel, sports, hanging out with friends, etc. As a culture, we are all faced with unpacking what life looks like in a world that is very different from what we thought it should be. Some of us are experiencing a collective cultural trauma in its infancy, and that can be a lot for a teen to unpack considering normal adolescent developmental pressures.

This book is designed to provide you with a brief understanding of the psychological, emotional, cultural, and spiritual considerations, framed in such a way that you can better support yourself and your teens. Don't worry, there is no need to have a degree in psychology in order to understand or support your teen's mental health. You don't need to have achieved optimal mental health yourself or have healed all your own past traumas, although you'll be challenged to look at them in order to remain accountable to yourself and to your teen.

What you do need is the desire to connect deeply and relate with an open mind and an open heart. This means dropping the story of who you think your teens should be and allowing them to be exactly who they are in this moment. This is the precise juncture where you will connect with them. This book will give you the tools, philosophy, science, and personal stories of healing to do just that. Even if you aren't close now, you can change that by first understanding the normal ups and downs of adolescence and transforming your perspective to create a deeper partnership with your teens. It is possible. It is worth the work. Remember, within families, relationships are the agent of change. Through connection, we heal.

Partnership Parenting

You will find the reference to "partnership parenting" and "partnership parenting paradigm" throughout this book. In fact, Chapter 4 is dedicated entirely to diving deeper into the underlying principles. It's not a term that is (yet) commonly found within the standard lexicon of our culture, but you will find references to partnership parenting in radical unschooling circles and those who are focused on conscious parenting, as well as within "hand-in-hand" parenting.

At this juncture, it is important to define what partnership parenting is and what it is not. Partnership parenting is approaching parenting through the lens of kindness, fairness, and partnership. This means approaching everything through the lens of equality and recognizing when you are slipping into the role of an authoritarian parent and out of the role of a partner or mentor. This includes recognizing your issues, beliefs, and fears surrounding control, bodily autonomy, consent, and respect among others.

The dominant culture has fed most of us the message over and over that "parents know best." We have been led to believe that our will, our perception of how children or teens should behave, is what is important. We have been programmed through years of messaging to believe it is our job to raise our children to be the kind of people we want them to be. Because we inherently believe we know what is best for them, we feel empowered to force, manipulate, or guilt them into doing what we want.

Answer this: Have you ever replied to your child or teen, "Because I'm the parent" or "Because I said so"?

I know I have heard those words come out of my mouth, and my parents have said the same thing to me in my own childhood countless times. Most of us were raised within an authoritarian parenting paradigm and are accustomed to authoritarian approaches within our culture. Most of us have accepted that tough love is needed at times and believe it's okay to impose our will on our children when it's for their benefit.

Most accept the authority imposed upon us through laws, cultural and societal guidelines, and rules found and practiced within the traditional education system. For most of us, we duplicate similar laws, guidelines, and rules within our own family structures.

Being raised in a culture where the underclass of people with the least amount of rights are children, most never introduce the idea of consent or equality into that relationship. If we think about it, most rules, bedtimes, restrictions, and expectations are arbitrary. Partnership parenting challenges this framework and looks at each individual as a capable and autonomous human being with the ability to self-regulate.

Are you getting triggered yet?
Maybe you are in the camp who is thinking, *I do not treat my teen through an authoritarian voice. I identify as a peaceful parent.* Authoritarian parenting doesn't always resemble a drill sergeant. It can also look like

coddling. The main component is to recognize that the parent is serving an agenda to control or manipulate their child in some manner. By doing this, we are not allowing our teens to have the experience to know or value their own autonomy and find their intrinsic motivation.

You might be saying at this moment, "But my teen is so lazy, they don't want to do ANYTHING! I have to manipulate them and demand them to do things, or they'll sleep all day!" We look at this myth a little deeper in Chapter 3, but there are strategies to partner with your teen based on shared values versus the sheer force of your will.

Recognize this. You were motivated to pick up this book to help facilitate your teen, so you must have the desire to support them in becoming happy and functioning adults. **After all, that's what all parents want.** The biggest difference between a partnership approach and authoritarian parenting is that the former encourages your teen to practice and experience accountability in a safe space, where making mistakes is part of the learning process and is expected. If your teen has never had the opportunity to experience accountability, which leads to self-regulation, you're not optimally preparing your teen to enter adulthood.

Considering how important developing the skills to care for and manage one's own mental health and emotional well-being is, you don't want to approach this topic through coercion. If you do, you run the risk of your teen creating a negative relationship with self-inquiry, which ultimately defeats the purpose of this book. I understand this is a lot to think about, and that, as parents, we must approach this with care and balance. But if we truly want to support our teens, I implore you to at least consider a partnership approach.

Now, let's look at this from the flip side. If we empower our teens to become accountable, as in all true partnerships, we too are accountable for our role in the relationship. As parents, we will need to be accountable for our triggers, reactions, dismissals, judgments, and expectations, which are oftentimes a result of our own childhood traumas. This is something we will explore deeper in Chapter 5.

Some of you may be reading this and thinking, *I picked up this book so I can help my teen change, not change myself!* Yes, but through partnership, there is equal accountability for changing what doesn't work, even if that is ourselves. The other aspect of change is that through partnership we don't get to decide what, if any, changes occur, as it is not our place to apply an agenda or manipulate someone else's behavior or development.

One of the last things I want to say about the partnership parenting paradigm is that you don't need to be perfect. Just considering a new way of being with your teen will help you to create a deeper and greater connection. If you decide ultimately this type of parenting is not for you, that's still okay. Keep this information in your mind and ask yourself within your challenging parenting moments, "Am I applying my own agenda to my teen's life in order to get the results I want? Am I dismissing my teen or implying what they are saying is not important because I don't agree, find it unworthy, ridiculous, or unimportant?" Then ask yourself, "How would this make me feel if my adult partner did this to me?"

Comfort Zone

When you're ready for a change, but it would require you to step out of your comfort zone, so you're just sitting there like

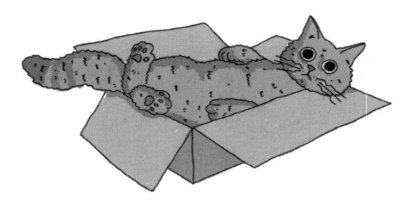

Within the work I do with teens, through both international travel experiences and my mentoring practice, comfort zone concepts are vital to creating familiar dialogue around current life experiences. Also, normalizing this topic among teens requires self-inquiry, and I urge parents to make this a common topic they talk about with their teens.

Often, this concept introduces teens to a new way to reflect on their life experiences, recognize the difference between inside-the-comfort-zone and outside-the-comfort-zone experiences, and have some clarity about their own lives, triggers, and limits. I often challenge teens to become aware of their own beliefs around being uncomfortable, unpack their individual meanings surrounding the topic, and look at the consequences in a new light.

Please don't underestimate the power of learning the tool below.

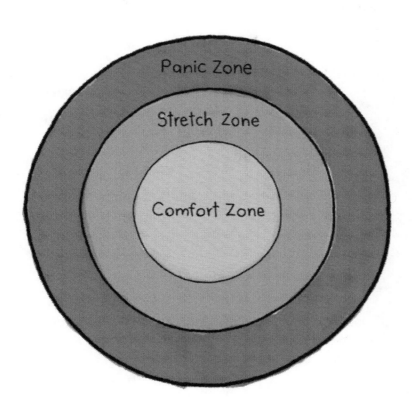

Briefly stated, the comfort zone is a state or situation in which one feels comfortable and is absent of anything new or difficult. Like a familiar embrace, our comfort zones can be both positive and equally confining. It is often the place from which we recuperate and regenerate. But it can also inhibit growth.

For most, the comfort zone is commonly perceived as a neutral space, but for some who have experienced traumas, the comfort zone may become a protective and isolating place to retreat to. Most of us can easily identify what things feel within our comfort zones without much of a problem. Many of us are conditioned to believe our comfort zone is the optimal space to be

45

and choose the comfort zone over the stretch zone. The purpose of this book is to challenge you to reconsider this thought.

Stretch Zone

The stretch zone is a place where learning or cortical mapping (the organizing of sensory inputs within the brain's cortex) happens, sparked through exploration and experiences. Until around age twenty-five, the adolescent brain is very plastic and is constantly making new neural connections by absorbing information, making sense of the world, and giving meaning to experiences. For teens, this is also a space where self-regulation starts to develop. Teens are wired to take risks, a topic we'll unpack in greater detail in Chapter 5.

But as you start to get into this book, I invite you to reflect on your own life, especially your adult life. Think about the times you've been outside of your comfort zone and you've immediately turned away from that experience. I'm sure you can think of a few. It is common within Western culture to avoid being uncomfortable. In fact, much of our adult lives are spent creating opportunities to avoid hardship, discomfort, or unease. This carries over into how we raise our children to look at the same obstacles and challenges.

Instead of recognizing discomfort as an indicator that we are growing, expanding, and learning, many adults respond to the discomfort by looking for ways to alleviate the uncomfortable sensations. At times, our responses to discomfort can look like medicating, numbing out, turning up the air conditioner when we are only slightly warm, or turning to distraction to help us avoid the sensations. Oftentimes, these are habits we've practiced since childhood, which were reinforced through a culture that automates, sanitizes, strives for optimal comfort, and creates remedies to not feel uncomfortable.

This is such a big topic.

Panic Zone

Let's take another look at the diagram. We are all familiar with the comfort zone. We just explored the stretch zone, and now we should briefly look at the panic zone. In Chapter 6, we will be further exploring the brain as it applies to our teens' development, but I wanted to touch on this briefly here as we look at the panic zone.

Most know the term "the reptilian brain," which was derived in the 1960s from Paul MacLean who defined the Triune Brain theory. In MacLean's model, the oldest part of the brain is known as the reptilian brain, which developed in animals over 100 million years ago. The main function of the primal-reptilian brain is to take care of our own survival by unconsciously acting instinctively. This part of the brain is lightning fast, automatic, and focused on our survival. The reptilian brain controls the involuntary systems of the body (breathing, heartbeat, organ function, body temperature), and it's also responsible for triggering our fight, flight, and freeze responses.

Our reptilian brain gets scared or angry very quickly, is territorial and aggressive, and can hold us in a state of anxiety. The reptilian brain works in conjunction with the amygdala, which asks the question, "Am I safe?" If the reptilian brain determines the answer is no, the amygdala goes offline, sometimes referred to as "flipping the lid," as we will explore in Chapter 6 with Dr. Daniel Siegel's hand model of the brain.

When the reptilian brain takes over, all the other systems go dormant, and survival mode is activated. It's important to note that the brain stem, the reptilian brain system, is designed to come online, block the danger through immediate action, then go back offline. Unfortunately, due to the heightened fear the world is experiencing currently, many young people have prolonged activation in this brain system, which is causing increased stress and anxiety.

Learning, Resilience & Change (Neuroplasticity)

We are going to talk about neuroplasticity in much greater detail as it pertains to the adolescent brain in Chapter 6, but it is important to understand how it relates to our personal development as adults and parents.

Neuroplasticity is simply the brain's neural network's ability to change through growth and reorganization. These changes range from individual neuron pathways making new connections, to systematic adjustments like cortical remapping. The term "neuroplasticity" came into the popular lexicon through Carol S. Dweck's seminal book *Mindset, The New Psychology of Success.*

Dweck writes about the differences between a fixed mindset and a growth mindset. In essence, they are defined as such:

- Fixed mindset: people believe their basic qualities, like their intelligence or talent, are simply fixed traits.
- Growth mindset: people believe their most basic abilities can be developed.

Which do you think is within the comfort zone experience?

If you answered, "a fixed mindset," you are right! A fixed mindset is within the comfort zone, and the growth mindset lies somewhere within the stretch zone. Since learning takes place outside the comfort zone, learning to embrace the discomfort of growth is really part of our work as parents.

Over the years, I've had hundreds of conversations with parents, friends, and former romantic partners about this topic. I've heard from numerous parents and partners who believe their personality is set or fixed: they know who they are, and it's impossible to change. I've heard this more times than I wish to admit and understand that change is an "inside job." I urge you to consider the following excerpt from Dweck's book mentioned earlier:

> Mindsets are an important part of your personality, but you can change them. Just by knowing about the two mindsets, you can start thinking and reacting in new ways. People tell me that they start to catch themselves when they are in the throes of the fixed mindset — passing up a chance for learning, feeling labeled by a failure, or getting discouraged when something requires a lot of effort. And then they switch themselves into the growth mindset — making sure they take the challenge, learn from the failure, or continue their effort.

Are you still wondering what mindset has to do with neuroplasticity? As described above, neuroplasticity is the ability to relearn or biologically rewire our brains to new patterns of thinking.

In essence, the first twenty-five years of a human's life lays down the wiring, determining how the brain processes and the meaning we give to our experiences. This cortical mapping is what we refer to as learning (or programming) which informs how we perceive both the outer worlds (perception) and inner worlds (interoception). In addition to many other processes the brain is responsible for, we are specifically addressing cortical mapping relating to perceptions, feelings, thoughts, behaviors, reactions, and translations of experiences into meaning.

During the first twenty-five years of development, the brain is pretty much plastic, learning freely, and forming new neural networks based on input. Learning during childhood and adolescence pretty much happens both actively and passively. However, for us adults after twenty-five, passive neuroplasticity is greatly reduced as our patterning is pretty much set. Okay, some of my former partners were correct.

In fact, as adults, the brain produces chemical processes which are activated when we try to consciously modify thought patterns, beliefs, perceptions, or behaviors. These chemicals make us uncomfortable because the brain is resisting change. But if we can recognize the brain is trying to preserve itself, we can welcome the uncomfortable feelings and choose to step into the stretch zone.

The good news is scientists have determined that neuroplasticity, or rewriting your beliefs, is available to all throughout our lifetime. For adult parents, neuroplasticity is possible. In other words, we can change how we view ourselves, how we view our children, and how we parent. But it's not comfortable.

As adults, we can change our thoughts because of neuroplasticity, but recognizing this requires two other processes:
- Intentional focus
- Rest or downtime to rewire our thinking

Parents, this is where your work comes in. This is why getting comfortable being uncomfortable is an essential sensation to recognize as you move through this book. I promise to make you uncomfortable with these words and many more going forward.

Commit Now to Becoming the Watcher

You might be asking yourself right now, "What is the watcher, and what exactly does it watch?" The watcher is the watcher of your thoughts and, as such, is responsible for observing your habitual thinking, especially when this thinking affects the way you see the world or interpret your teen's behavior. These thoughts nudge you to coerce your teen or apply an agenda. This takes practice though, and throughout this book, you'll find strategies to support your teen through greater self-inquiry. You too are responsible for developing that muscle.

For you, your work as a parent facilitator within the partnership parenting paradigm is to uncover the belief systems you've been practicing throughout your life, which determines how you parent, where the ideas you have for "proper" behavior come from, and what agendas you live out through your interactions. This is your wiring, your programming, and the stuff you are accountable for, especially as it affects the interaction between you and your teen. In essence, you cannot support your teen if you are trying (consciously or unconsciously) to manipulate your teen to fulfill a particular agenda.

I'm not going to lie – this is tough work. We'll get into this deeper within the pages of this book, but start practicing by listening to the voice of the thinker and becoming the watcher who listens.

Self-Directed Learning

"If education is going to be transformative, it's going to be uncomfortable and unpredictable."
                                                            ~ Brené Brown

As I described in the intro of this book, I am a proud self-directed learner. I also raised a self-directed learner. This style of education is often referred to as unschooling, child-led education, independent study, parent-supported learning, natural learning, autodidactism, life-long learning, or worldschooling. Even though all of these have slightly nuanced approaches and philosophies, the constant thread between these approaches is that the learner is in charge of guiding their educational pursuits.

The reason an entire subsection of this chapter is dedicated to self-directed learning is for you, the parent. The intention is not to convince you to modify your adolescent's educational approach, but rather to empower you as a self-directed learner, who is driving your own learning about yourself, your teen's experience, and the relationship between the two. You can support and facilitate your teen's mental health journey by increasing your understanding and knowledge and placing your experiences into context around these topics. That's why you are reading this book, right?

Over the past decades, many education scholars and psychology researchers have focused on studying the importance of self-directed learning in adults. In an academic paper entitled *Learning in Adulthood: A Comprehensive Guide,* the authors Merriam, Caffarella, and Baumgartner have described three main goals for adult self-directed learning. These goals are referenced throughout this book:

1. Enhancing the ability of learners to be self-determined
2. Fostering transformational learning
3. Promoting emancipatory learning and social action.

Throughout these pages, you will find ways to enhance your learning, transform old beliefs, and encourage action. You will be empowered through a variety of valuable information, resources, support, and inspiration. We've got this!

For those of you who are already involved in the unschooling movement, some of these concepts will not be new to you. The idea of facilitation, partnership, guiding, and getting out of the learner's way are all parts of the foundation of self-directed learning. For those of you just being introduced to this modality of education, there is a comprehensive Suggested Reading section at the back of this book with many useful resources on this topic. Those of you not interested at all, that's fine too!

Deschooling

Within the unschooling community, we often refer to the process of changing your beliefs about the nature of education as "deschooling." This literally means noticing when the old beliefs come up, unlearning those beliefs, questioning their validity, and deciding if they still serve you. If we decide they do not, we must consciously replace them with new beliefs in alignment with the values intrinsic to directing one's own education. As long as you didn't grow up under a rock, every single one of us has been exposed to a lifetime of normative cultural beliefs surrounding education, teens, parenting, and how the world should run. Deschooling in self-directed education circles dives into the myth that a good education is the approved path to learning anything important, and you will be rewarded with a happy life and the promise of financial well-being.

Most of us have been convinced that in order to achieve this promise, we must put our learning in the hands of those who know best: teachers, professors, and institutions. This message runs through the dominant culture, and most of us never question it.

What if I told you this was a lie? What if I told you this is one of the most disempowering pieces of fiction told and retold throughout our culture? What if I told you all you need is to be empowered through tools and the confidence to use them? What if I said you can support your teen in a journey into the depths of self? What comes up in you? Are you feeling frightened, defensive, or triggered?

In the context of this book, the old ideas you are faced with questioning may sound like: "teens are impulsive," "teens are rude," "teens are rebellious," and many other similar beliefs. In fact, we dedicate an entire chapter to dispelling those cultural teen myths in Chapter 3.

One of the greatest deschooling challenges you may face when moving through this book is believing you can learn enough to start healing yourself. I know you can integrate and understand your childhood wounds, which created belief systems and patterns of behavior that have influenced how you view your teen. Oftentimes, these old patterns you are carrying with you lead to harmful and unreasonable expectations of your children. You can self-direct your own discovery into these spaces. You can be equipped to support and effectively facilitate your teen's mental health journey.

The connection between self-directed learning and self-directed healing is much the same. The self-directed learning journey taps into the learner's intrinsic motivation to learn, dig deeper, and transform their understanding. The self-directed healing journey takes the learning and adds an element of self-inquiry and conscious and unconscious integration.

Tools of Facilitation

What is facilitation, and how is it different from teaching?

Great question!

Before you try to use any of the tools shared throughout this book, it's imperative you can distinguish those differences. The information and tools presented here are not meant for you to teach your teen, rather they are provided to prepare you with a deeper understanding of *why* tools can be beneficial to supporting mental health and *how* to use them. There are subtle differences between teaching and facilitating these tools, and I will briefly attempt to describe those differences here using philosophy borrowed from the foundations of unschooling (self-directed learning).

The first and most important point of differentiation is that facilitation relies on trust and respect over fear and control. Which set of attributes do you think the traditional educational model uses?

Let's first examine what facilitation is not.

When rewards or punishments are associated with an activity, when coercion is present, and when there is an unequal balance of power; this is an authoritarian model and not facilitation. When a person demands a learner participate in expectation of a particular result, they are not facilitating. When a person asserts power, controls the process, and uses manipulation to achieve a certain outcome, this is not facilitation.

Facilitation happens through partnership, and facilitation must engage consent.

Let's think back to when your adolescent was a young child, just learning to walk. They learned to walk and initiated that process by themselves as a natural extension of growing and developing. You didn't need to manipulate or control the process. Your role was very easy, natural, and instinctual. I am certain you did not sit your child down, pull out biology books, make them study the muscle structure, practice leg extensions, or test them on the theory of balancing or weight distribution concepts. Even as a toddler, if they could understand lessons of that type, they would still begin to walk when they were ready, no matter what you tried to teach them. If they were not ready to walk, no lesson or coercion could make them walk, no matter how much you demanded.

I bet you can remember those first steps, chubby arms and legs shaking, muscle control developing as they tried to pull themselves upright. The shaking legs were learning balance and often resulted in landing on that squishy bottom. You likely watched attentively, your arms spread around the outer perimeter making sure your child's path was safe.

You were there. You didn't demand they walk when they weren't ready. You allowed them to work out their weight distribution, supported them so they felt safe, and allowed the experience to unfold. You facilitated their natural experience of learning, and you didn't teach them a contrived choreographed sequence of steps to mimic. Your acute instinct guided you to allow and trust your baby's steps to unfold. You were the perfect facilitator, and your facilitation was likely as natural as breathing.

Remember what it felt like to support and help your child when they are ready. Access the patience and deep-flowing love you had in those moments. You'll need to keep this model in mind as you are ready to approach, partner, and facilitate your teen with the tools from this book.

Another subtle aspect of facilitating is through modeling. Modeling is not teaching. It is showing, sharing, connecting, and living the experience you'd like to support your child to learn. In the case of the toddler learning to walk, you modeled what walking looked like by being your authentic walking self. By naturally doing what you normally do, you supported them on their journey into becoming a walker.

Unlike walking, facilitating mental health practices will require a little more intentionality. In the case of facilitating these tools, you as the parent will need to use the tools on yourself first and share with your teen the discoveries revealed through your own journey. That requires trust and willingness to share vulnerability in order to create greater connection and trust, one of the key elements required to facilitate work of this nature.

Facilitation can take many forms. In unschooling communities, parents are urged to pay attention to their children's areas of interest. Facilitating children in the unschooling world looks like providing resources, suggesting websites and books, watching movies on those topics together, and engaging in conversation.

Facilitating teens is not as straightforward since we must recognize adolescence is a time of individuation, directed in part by biological development. However, you likely picked up this book because you were concerned about some aspect of your teen's mental health, and that's the place you can start engaging in meaningful conversations now. Let them know you are learning, processing your own inner workings, and practicing using tools in order to support them better. Invite them to ask questions and learn about your discoveries in the spirit of being the best facilitator you can be for them on their current journey.

Sharing is an important aspect of facilitation. In the case your teen isn't interested, ready, or willing to know more, not all is lost. If you commit to going deeper within yourself, it will affect the relationships around you without any coercion. By examining, uncovering, healing, and creating greater awareness of your own inner workings, you can't help but create a beacon of light for your teen, thus creating the space to connect, where perhaps your teen hadn't noticed it before.

Part of the facilitator's role is to authentically share the learner's enthusiasm and support them with genuine interest. This creates a greater connection and a closer attached relationship. Where the unschooling philosophy may fall short is overlooking an intentional culture of reciprocation, which is inherent within a partnership parenting paradigm. As part of the culture of raising your adolescent, you must strive for connection, which is at the core of facilitation. Even if your teen is pulling away, the path to connection is through your willingness to be vulnerable and share with your teen. Facilitation is a two-person dance, and sometimes as the adult, we need to take a step back, re-establish the connection, do some relationship repair work, and show up authentic and vulnerable without expectation or coercion. It's a delicate dance for sure.

Another key aspect of facilitation borrowed from unschooling philosophy is the strategy to meet your child in his or her learning field. Be mindful of what comes up as you start deprogramming or deschooling your own beliefs about your teen. Noticing when you are seeing your teen through the lens of judgment is vital to the process.

You will be triggered by your teen's behavior at times. That is your opportunity to use these tools to actively question your programmed expectations of your teen, check your limiting beliefs, and commit to this process. If not, those expectations will not allow you to facilitate without an agenda, and that agenda is an act of coercion. This is the work in the facilitation-partnership you are solely accountable for. I am offering you the *how* through the exercises and tools found in later chapters. But the big unspoken *how* is committing to your process too.

Another facilitation strategy can be found in taking your teen's questions seriously. This can be difficult for you when the topic is uncomfortable and/or the timing is inconvenient. Notice if you have an immediate reaction within you that pushes you into a state of judgment. Judgment will shut down the connection at a second's notice. Facilitating is the ability within you to cultivate your skills to be able to take your teen's questions as far as they want to go. Make sure you follow their lead and create space for them to be seen, heard, and understood without judgment. Facilitating is also cultivating the skill to recognize and honor when your teen stops responding and knowing when it's your time to step back. It's subtle, but you can learn to recognize this.

Finally, facilitating requires being present. Being available to your teen can be the most difficult aspect of this journey. I know you have so much to do, many worries, and much to manage. We all want a quick fix and the perfect road map, but recognize from this point forward, it's messy, time-consuming, uncomfortable, and not terribly efficient. But it's also unbelievably rewarding to connect, facilitate, and partner with your teen.

Managing Your Expectations

I just wrote about expectations in the context of facilitation. But before moving forward, I have to briefly address how you must manage your own expectations throughout this process. First and foremost, you must accept this process will be slow and expect change to happen gradually. You must commit to the process through a willingness to examine your own "stuff" AND be open and transparent throughout.

If you are seeking a set of tools to simply apply and fix your teen, I recommend you put this book down right now. That is not here. Rather, expect to be guided through creating a new lifelong relationship with mental health.

This is an invitation to redefine your understanding of what mental health is. Many believe mental health focuses on fixing a specific problem. Although managing anxiety, depression, or changing behavior may be the goal of immediate mental health practices, mental health is not an achievement, where the work ends once you arrive.

Think about a person who is exercising or dieting solely with the intent to lose weight. In most cases, this is not the optimal mindset. Within this approach, the person measures their success through a specific result. Those who manage to reach a weight goal don't tend to keep the weight off.

Now, consider the approach or mindset of the person who is committed to living healthy. Dieting and exercise may be one of the things they do, but they don't stop the moment the scale hits a magical number. They maintain a healthy lifestyle by committing to themselves and using tools. This is how I suggest you approach your own mental health and your teen's.

In essence, managing your own expectations may require a change in perception and understanding that mental health is not a destination or an achievement. It is a lifelong process worthy of your attention. Your mental health literacy will add to your teen's experience, but the process of awareness will have to start with you from exactly where you are right now.

Teens in a Time of Change

Beyond just the normal challenges of adolescence, times of change can be especially difficult for teens. When the ground beneath us does not feel steady, many of us get stuck on the Trauma Train. Teens are wired to start stepping out into greater independence but have a more difficult time doing so when they feel unsafe or when there are overwhelming restrictions prohibiting them to do so, based on circumstances beyond their control.

The current generation may not yet be able to articulate how this new reality is affecting them. Most children grow up idealizing the time in their lives when they become a teenager and, in one way or another, are excited about having new paths to choose and stepping into greater independence. Western culture idolizes these years through countless coming-of-age movies, pop culture memes, and the high school social experience narrative. However, we find ourselves in a time in history that conflicts with these social expectations as a result of this global pandemic. This is especially more challenging for the older adolescents, as they were poised to launch into independence and now find themselves, pardon the expression, "screwed" with a lack of options. The older teens I've been working with experience a greater sense of despair, knowing they have limited options preventing them from moving out of their parents' home, finding summer jobs, being restricted from traveling freely, and facing tighter economic options. Even the college experience is not what they expected, filled with restrictions and, in many cases, virtual classrooms. This can lead to greater depression and uncertainty about the future, more than they already had to begin with.

The pandemic has forced us to be more conscious than ever about how our teens function in periods of extreme stress or change, and that is not necessarily a bad thing. The United States Center for Disease Control reported that hospitalizations amongst teens for mental health reasons spiked by 31% in 2020. Suicide attempts spiked in young women by a staggering 50.6%. States such as California reported a dramatic increase of deaths in minors from suicide, in the hundreds of percentiles. We are seeing the effects of uncertainty on our youth, and this is something we cannot ignore.

From the parent's perspective (yes, I'm talking to you), please don't try to solve this problem for your adolescent– you can't. You need to be conscious of what is going on and share those frustrations with your teens to help validate their unspoken fears. This will bridge that parental-authority gap, slip into greater partnership, and help to build a healthy, strong connection.

Chapter 3: Teen Myths

The familiar feeling of heaviness surrounds my heart and stomach, sinking inward until my body collapses into itself. This is how it always starts. Then, the heat penetrates my back, rises up to my neck to the top of my head, then ascends down across my forehead into my cheeks. Then, my eyes automatically drop to the ground, and they start to fill with tears as my chest and stomach collapse deeper into myself. This is what shame feels like to me, and how it manifests in my body. This is something I felt a lot growing up.

My experience as a child and a teen was filled with constant violations. "But you can't be trusted," my mother would say, excusing her constant intrusion into my room. She said she needed to make sure my room was in order, things were in their place, clothes folded and put away, and God forbid, no "garbage" in the waste-paper basket. I'd often come home from school with piles of clothes on the center of my bedroom floor that I had earlier hastily shoved into my closet. "Do it right, or don't do it at all," I could hear my mother's words. In my mind, I wanted to respond, "Then I won't do it at all," but that was never an option. Not only was that never an option, but neither was talking back to her.

There were times I'd returned from school to find the trash cans emptied onto my bedroom floor when there were items placed there that did not align with the rigid house rules. Other times, I'd find my bed torn apart to be remade if the bed hadn't been previously made to my mother's liking. Unfortunately, my childhood was filled with incidents like these, not isolated and with too many examples to recount.

The biggest feeling of violation occurred when I entered adolescence. My mother began to read my diary no matter how many places I tried to hide it: in my closet, under my mattress, or behind a stack of books on my bookshelves. She always found it. At first, I thought I was going mad. I'd come home from school to find my diary placed in the middle of my bed. With a puzzled look, I'd ask myself, "Could I have left it out?" At first, I really wasn't sure. My mom would say nothing, just give me a knowing look, always resulting in the familiar feeling of violation and shame washing over my body.

Soon I came to know it wasn't my imagination. It was not safe to commit my innermost thoughts, fears, and doubts to the pages of my diary because I knew they were not protected or private. I responded by asserting the only power I could think of; I started to write fictional stories about doing drugs and recorded the numerous hiding places I discovered in my room that my mother could never uncover. Then, in all the hiding places mentioned in my diary, I'd place a variety of messages on tiny pieces of paper, saying things like, "F*ck you, Mom, I hate you!" My mother never said anything, but the notes mysteriously vanished from their hiding places.

Ironically, my mother's intrusions did not protect me from doing drugs, having sex, or any of the other behaviors she proclaimed she was so worried about. In fact, her style of parenting drove me towards those things to a greater degree, which oftentimes reflected in some pretty destructive decision-making.

Overall, I felt ashamed of who I was, and throughout my entire adolescence, I had never experienced the feeling of safety. Not feeling safe was something that bled through to my early adult relationships as well and prevented me from being fully trusting, until I focused on healing those traumas, which turned into forming new beliefs many years later.

It's easy to read the research on the teenage brain and come up with generalizations about adolescents, concluding that teenagers are irrational, loose cannons who can't be trusted. Maybe they can; maybe they can't. But there are many factors to consider, like the experience of the teen's home life, brain development (of course), and beliefs teens have created about themselves.

My adolescence was riddled with many of the behaviors we are going to explore in this chapter of myths. What looked like teen rebellion for me was really a cry for connection. I urge you to consider that these behaviors and myths are not created in a vacuum, and if you recognize any of these things in your teen, please explore what needs may not be met from your teen's perspective.

Teens Are Impulsive

This myth isn't untrue, but it has more to do with biology than teens simply making bad choices or being "impulsive." Impulsivity in teens is actually a biological response.

During adolescence, the prefrontal cortex is not completely developed and does not come totally online until about the age of twenty-five. This is the area of the brain credited with helping humans process consequences, among other things. Many scientific studies show cognitive control and emotion regulation improves with maturation from childhood into adulthood.

The teenage brain is influenced by the neurotransmitter dopamine very differently than its adult counterparts. Neurotransmitters are the body's chemical messengers, which have a direct correlation with our moods. Dopamine is the "happy" neurotransmitter, and everyone on the planet feels happier when they experience a dopamine release. During adolescence, the brain produces an enhanced dopamine supply and grows more receptors, which provides a rush that adults don't feel when engaged in the same activity.

Because of the happiness or pleasure felt with this process, the brain's reward system can override warning signals about risk in young people. This doesn't mean teens don't know better or are not capable of stopping to consider the consequences. To some degree, it's just not an automatic and natural response. I'd venture to guess that teens have some idea of what *could* happen, but the feeling that the risk may totally be worth it outweighs the consequence. We should reframe the myth that "teens are impulsive" to "teens have a lack of brakes."

Dr. Daniel Siegel, author of *Brainstorm: The Power and Purpose of the Teenage Brain,* makes the argument that the reason adolescence is vital to humanity's survival is because this stage is filled with the most ingenuity, courage, and creativity, which can change the course of humanity. Considering thousands of years ago when the average lifespan was much shorter than it is today, adolescents were in the prime of their lives and looked to as soldiers, hunters, and heads of household.

The flip side of an elevated dopamine release within the adolescent brain is the preexistence of hyperrationality, which we'll explore in greater detail in Chapter 6. With hyper-rational thinking, we fail to see the big picture and miss the setting or context of the situation. It also supports the fixation on one part of the experience, likely the benefits, and totally ignores the potential consequences.

Knowing your teen's brain works differently than your adult brain, it's your duty to empower your teens by educating them so that you can better support them. So, while they may be more impulsive-acting, we can help our teens to see their blind spots through compassionate communication and even celebrate the process together. If a bad decision does arise, it's our job to support, not shame, connect, and explore the nonpunitive natural consequences that arise as a result.

Teens Are Lazy

Teens sleep all hours of the day, stay up late, and are completely content with doing nothing all day. They are just naturally lazy beings, right?

Wrong. Consider this, **the teenage mind is a very busy place**. There are lots of things going on. In fact, the teenage brain is going through a process called remodeling.

Remodeling in the brain is a necessary part of adolescent development and includes two biological features.

First, remodeling involves synaptic pruning. Pruning is when the brain determines which neural pathways, from our experiences from birth until this point, are valid and necessary. These neural pathways were created from our lifetime of experiences and contain thoughts, memories, emotions, and information about ourselves and the world around us. The brain determines which information is important to us and which neural pathways are not. Those that are not then get pruned away.

The second aspect of remodeling is called myelination. Myelination is the process by which an electrically-insulated layer known as a myelin sheath develops over the brain's neurons. This myelin sheath allows the neurocircuitry in the teen brain to strengthen, promoting greater multitasking and enhancing the ability to solve problems and the capability to process complex information. The process also increases the resting time between neural firings, which helps the brain to work optimally.

Sometimes during the remodeling process, teens can experience challenges as new ways of thinking, feeling, and interacting are being defined. In reality, the remodeling process is energy-consuming.

Another consideration to the "teens are lazy" myth is the natural changes in their sleep habits. This is explained by the naturally occurring hormone our body produces called melatonin. When it gets dark, the hypothalamus sends a message to the pineal gland to increase the production of melatonin, and we are alerted it's time to get some rest. As melatonin levels rise, we feel more and more sleepy. After we've gotten sufficient rest, our melatonin levels dip, and we wake up. Simple, right?

Well, as nature would have it, puberty triggers a change in this cycle. Young people experience melatonin surges later at night, and melatonin dips later in the morning. Falling asleep early can be rare, and the desire to sleep in later is natural.

What do you think, are teens really lazy or are they just exhausted as an effect of all the biological changes?

Teens Are Rude

This is a blanket statement that is no truer for adults. Sometimes people are just downright rude, but a teen is not wired to be rude just because of their age. Remember, there is a lot of change going on in their heads at a rapid rate, and it could be quite overwhelming. Their reactions may not necessarily be driven by the person they are speaking to but rather by learning how to identify and use the tools at their disposal. And sometimes hyper-rational thinking can be expressed through one-word responses or even that "look." (You know the one.)

Teens who are not actively engaged in inner-discovery work may be less likely to recognize their triggers and go into reaction mode instead of consciously responding. This takes practice, and that's why you are reading this book.

Parenting A Teen Is Hard

Parents ultimately want what is best for their kids, right? However, we, as parents, fall into the trap of making three main mistakes with our teens: 1.) placing expectations on them 2.) controlling them, and 3.) dismissing their needs, wants, or desires.

Here's what you need to know: Expectations are relationship killers. All expectations come from the misguided belief that we are right. After all, we've already been through our teen years, right? However, parents can be blind to the influence of their own unhealed traumas, triggers, and beliefs, which is a topic we'll explore in greater detail throughout this book. When the parent isn't aware of what is going on in their own subconscious experience, it's literally impossible to be open and objective. The reality is, as parents impose their will on their teens, even if it's with the best of intentions, our teenagers will likely push back in some form or another.

Control does not bring connection. You cannot control your way into a relationship with your teen, you cannot control the state of their mental health or their behavior, nor can you control your teen to be more respectful or to become any other misguided desire you may be entertaining. Control is an action stemming from authoritarian parenting. Control is what my mother did throughout my entire childhood and adolescence. Control can irrevocably damage your relationship.

On the flip side of control, you'll find dismissal. Dismissing your teen is the opposite of helping your teen to feel safe, heard, seen, and understood. Their emotions, ideas, and concepts are important, even if they are different from your own. I know many families whose teens have opposing political beliefs. I know many teens who are shut down at the dinner table during conversations with their parents because they are told their opinion doesn't matter, they don't know what they are talking about, and the ideas they have are invalid.

Simply put, don't do this. Allow yourself to step into your own stretch zone and hear their thoughts, ideas, and values come through. Dismissing your teen is one of the most invalidating things you can do, and the damage to their self-esteem can run deep. How do I know? I lived in a state of constant dismissal.

Remember, just because you are the adult does not give you blanket authority over your teen, permission to control every decision in their lives, or an invitation to invade their privacy or dismiss their perspectives. It is ok if reading this makes you want to throw the book across the room— throw it! Then take a deep breath and pick it back up when you are ready but realize putting pressure on your kids does not help.

I'm not going to lie to you, parenting, in general, is hard. Each age has its own set of challenges but reframing the challenge into an honor can shift our perspective and approach. In other words, anything in life is as hard as we make it. The more we learn and adapt our behaviors and approach to meet teens where they are, the better the chances of ease and peace we will find.

Teen's Hormones Are Raging

Yes...but that's only half of the story. It's true, the body and mind of an adolescent are changing rapidly during this stage of life. Those changes were once exclusively accredited to the myth of raging hormones, but current research has uncovered a more complex set of biological changes. As we explored earlier, the teenage brain is indeed remodeling, but those changes are not as visible as the hormonal changes. In contrast, hormonal changes cause clear outward signs, and they are impossible to ignore.

Hormonal changes in an adolescent bring a set of physiological changes including:
- Growth spurts
- Increased sweating
- Acne
- Growth of pubic and armpit hair

One of the most obvious and challenging aspects of adolescence is developing sexual maturity. Teens become more aware of their sexuality, gender identity, and attraction preferences during adolescence, more than at any other phase of life. Commonly, the first sexual experience occurs during this period as well, so it's extremely important for parents to talk to their teens openly about the subject.

As if hormonal-physical changes weren't enough, the coinciding process of brain remodeling can also play havoc on the teen's emotional state. The remodeling brain can be experienced in varying degrees through the teen's emotional spark, desire for social engagement, relationship to novelty, and creative pursuits. Whoa, there's a lot going on!

The adolescent brain is filled with more emotional processes than during any other period of a person's development. Emotional sparks can be the reason teens experience moodiness, irritability, and an inability to trust their own emotional states. But on the other side of the coin, when things are good, life is on fire and can be fully charged with passion and purpose! During this stage, social engagement is super important.

Combine all of those overlapping mental and physical changes, and the result can be overwhelming for a teen. There is no manual available to provide a roadmap, but you can help to be their guide. What works for one person will not necessarily work for another. So as a supporting parent, creating dialogue around these transformations and helping teens understand what changes are going on inside of them may be the best way to support them.

Teens Are Immature

This is one of my favorite "myths," and I quote that because it is not so much the statement that is misguided, but the parental belief that teens should be expected to be totally mature and stop acting like a child. We don't make a baby feel bad for playing with its toys or a pre-teen for playing video games, so why do we expect a teen to automatically outgrow things they enjoy?

One of the leading authorities on the belief that teens learn and retain more when they are free to play is Dr. Peter Gray. I have had the honor of interviewing Dr. Gray multiple times on the principles he sets forth in his book *Free to Learn: Why Unleashing the Instinct to Play Will Make Our Children Happier, More Self-Reliant, and Better Students for Life*. He speaks extensively about the five elements that dictate what play is. An overview of each is below, but for more information, please go buy his book.

1. Play is self-chosen/self-directed: This is the social aspect where children learn how to negotiate. In this element, they explore how to get their needs met.
2. Play is intrinsically rewarding: When children play for the sake of playing, it's fun, and there's always learning involved.
3. Play always has rules: Yet they are rules the players opt into or create, which allows players to control their instincts and whims.
4. Play always has some element of imagination.
5. Play is conducted in a non-stress frame of mine, and players are free to quit.

To look at these through an instinctual lens, let's compare the evolutionary development of human beings to that of lion cubs. From the time lion cubs are born, they are constantly playing and roughhousing with each other. If one didn't know better, it might seem like there was a level of animosity at play, but it is just their primal way of testing the neural pathways that shape how they learn. Humans are not so different, with the possible exception of biting and scratching!

As parents, we tend to overschedule our kid's time with all the various activities they take part in, and it leaves very little time for free play. The groups of teens going to traditional school have the biggest issue with this because of all the other rules and structures they must abide by. This makes them the most susceptible to binging on video games and feeling compelled to complete everything being asked of them in the game.

Parents need to have a dialogue about this from a brain perspective and psychological perspective because the brain regulation function has not been fully developed in teens. Imagine sending someone into a boxing ring without any technical or endurance training– you'd be setting them up for failure! Teens have no natural ability to fully calculate risks and rewards due to the developing prefrontal cortex. This makes it very difficult for them to thrive. To facilitate their success, we must take into consideration all the physical and biological components that factor in.

Teens Are Addicted to Their Screens

Teens are addicted to their screens, phones, video games, and social media!

Parents must limit their teen's screen time for their own good!

How many times have you thought, said, or done this? Your belief may echo those of countless parents around the world in online teen support groups, parenting forums, and home education communities, all expressing concerns about their teen's screen time. Many worried parents stand firm in the belief that limiting screen time is essential because teens are addicted to gaming and social media, and they must have better things to do with their time.

But is this really true? You can absolutely find countless expert opinions arguing the dangers of screen addiction causing out-of-control social anxiety, poor self-image, and even depression. However, some experts believe playing video games, being active on social media, and excessive screen time is a way of coping with social anxiety, depression, and feeling of lack of control in one's life.

Let's first address screen time. Screens are obviously connected to computers, phones, and tablets. These devices lead to sources of information and are arguably one of the most important tools in modern society. Why would we limit our teen's opportunities to engage with information?

Most parents recognize how much the world has changed since they themselves were teenagers. Now, we all have devices that can fit into our pockets, keeping us connected to the world, our friends, entertainment, and news and providing a framework for understanding our culture. Now, especially in a time of COVID, teens need this connection, rather a lifeline, to the world around them.

This is not to say there are no issues surrounding dangerous content, unsafe social connections, or even access to unhealthy self-image messaging. All these things exist in the online world as they exist in the physical world. All these topics are the responsibility of the parent to discuss with their teen through connection, not coercion. Taking away their phone or limiting access to the internet will create a culture of secrecy, and those tough conversations will be difficult to have.

Many parents believe video game playing is addictive and often criticize their teens for playing. For a moment, think about this from the perspective of the teen, who has been told the very thing they value is useless, a waste of time. Think about the potential negative effects this conflict has on your teen and your relationship.

Your belief that video games are addictive may be at the root of this conflict. There is a distinction between gaming and other types of addictions. Both activate pleasure responses in the brain and encourage dopamine releases. However, substances, such as heavy drugs, create dependence on the chemical release, seeking a constant state of pleasure or numbing out. In contrast, video games require skills and perseverance as players overcome challenges and, in some cases, spend countless hours of research and play to achieve specific goals, thus resulting in gradual dopamine releases associated with achievement.

But let's recognize that this is not just present with video game playing. Any person who gains new skills, like learning a new song on a guitar, running a marathon they trained months for, or writing an epic poem, can also result in similar dopamine releases.

Dr. Peter Gray, the author of the book *Free to Learn,* approaches this subject slightly differently than other psychologists. There are unhealthy habits and scheduling problems, but according to Dr. Peter Gray, there are no addictions, especially when it comes to video games. According to Peter Gray, "Children aren't suffering today from too much computer play or screen time. They are suffering from too much adult control over their lives and not enough freedom."

Regardless of your belief, I am inviting you to look at this issue through a new lens and consider how you approach this topic in service of your relationship with your teen.

Teen Rebellion Is Bad

Yes, most teens will rebel. So how can this be a myth?

As with most of the other myths I've debunked, this one too is rooted within the biological, emotional, and psychological changes adolescents experience. Deep within all those changes, we can see the desire to individuate. In fact, one of the key tasks of the teenage years is to explore and discover their own identity. At the root of teenage rebellion, teen angst is a sign that they are trying new ways of looking at themselves and being in the world. In fact, the teen rebel is mislabeled and should be referred to as the "intrepid explorer."

So, if teenage rebellion is about exploring identities and individuating, is that really bad?

As parents, our work is to reframe the experience and understand their behavior from a new compassionate perspective. Does your son's black eyeliner really scream rebellion? Does their experimentation with different pronouns mean they are rebelling against your values? Does your teen's sudden disinterest in tennis mean she's rebelling against your family's traditions? Their choices to explore new ways of being may not actually be in opposition to you; it can simply be a new road they are traveling down, seeking to find themselves. In Chapter 5, I explore identities deeper including Jung's archetypes, which may help you understand identity formation. Teens may commit to new identities, beliefs, values, ambitions, careers, interests, or relationships you don't approve of.

This may be a part of their journey toward creating a robust sense of self. It is really your job to help your teen rebel successfully! Read that again. Constructive support looks like this:
- Encouraging your teen to ask hard questions
- Taking an interest in their pursuits and interests
- Encouraging open discussion about ideas and values without judgment
- Talking freely and clearly about your own values and decisions without judgment
- Accepting their choices without the need to prove anything

"Rebellion is when you look society in the face and say, 'I understand who you want me to be, but I'm going to show you who I actually am!'"
~Anthony Anaxagorou

Rebellion can also include the act of questioning everything! As annoying as this sounds, if you have a teen who naturally does this, please encourage more of this. If your teen does not question things, encourage them to try. This kind of exploration within the environment of your family culture means they feel safe to be seen, heard, and understood.

Finally, our greatest work in parenting a teen, especially during the uncomfortable stages, is to not take things personally. If we approach our teens in opposition to their choices, they may stubbornly over-identify with something, which might be a passing phase.

If you can, please look at the adolescence period through the lens of wonderment. There are many generalities that correlate with certain stages of development, and our culture tends to weave these changes into myths. Understand that historically this stage of development is very important to the individual and society as a whole. Political movements were born through adolescence idealism, as were great art and music. Adolescence prepares us to get ready to leave home, live as independent adults, and make our mark on the world. In order to do this, young people need to learn to take greater risks, think creatively, and seek the unfamiliar.

For parents, the experience of pedal-to-the-metal changes in your teen can be daunting. With the growing influence of peers, new friend groups, and new identities into the mix, many parents run for the hills. By putting all of these brain processes in a developmental context and learning to reframe your perspective, you too can challenge these myths and create your own understanding. Young people need many things during this stage. They need to be seen, heard, and understood, as well as have the freedom to somewhat enjoy the thrill of it all in order to complete an incredibly overwhelming task: **growing up**.

Chapter 4: Parenting A Teen

I was a fifteen-year-old runaway.

I couldn't stand the feeling anymore, the weight of being judged, the heaviness of being controlled, or the emptiness of not being seen, heard, or understood.

Before I left, I spent as much time away from the house as I could, with friends or my boyfriend or hanging out somewhere in my neighborhood. My mom worked some evenings, and the nights she wasn't home, I felt like I could exhale a little. The evenings she was in the home, it felt like a dense black hole of heavy energy, where I felt my value as a human being was reduced to utter nothinglessness.

Then, one day, something snapped. I was done. I couldn't take it anymore. I left.

My fifteen-year-old boyfriend and I devised a plan to leave both of our challenging home situations and took what became an almost six-month adventure.

At first, we stayed with friends. Then we moved into a seedy motel in the neighboring town. We took to selling drugs and, of course, we didn't go to school. A month later, I got my first job working as a waitress in a cafe, which I was pretty bad at, but the tips kept us going. We didn't make the best decisions, and when my boyfriend got arrested for robbery, I negotiated terms with my parents to return home.

However, what I learned about myself and the world was priceless. I discovered I was capable of immense strength through independence, which I later learned is a very common trauma response.

When I returned home again, things felt a little different. Although the relationship between me and my mother was not repaired, she learned to

75

back off a little, which made our lives together under the same roof a little more tolerable.

One of the conditions of my return home was that I had to go back to high school. I was enrolled in an alternative school, which employed an independent study program. Over the next six months, I managed to complete the few months of high school I had missed AND complete the equivalent of the next two years of high school. Everyone was shocked that I was a motivated, self-directed learner. I really saw it as a means to an end. With the combination of the credits, I earned and an equivalency exam, I graduated high school at sixteen years old and went off to college the next year.

"Let your past experiences serve as a reminder of your resilience rather than evidence of an unsafe world. Life isn't trying to break you down. it's trying to break you open."
~ Sheleana Aiyana

If you are reading this book, I suspect you are actively trying to avoid the kind of parenting I experienced during my childhood. However, even parents with the best of intentions can be left feeling bewildered and aware of their sudden lack of effectiveness when parenting the elusive adolescent. With everything we explored in Chapter 3, it might seem like parenting in the teen years is an impossible task. Throughout this chapter, I'll be exploring the strategies for parenting through the lens of connection, which is really the key to all of this.

Running away was my way of responding to the situation in my home life. What I was really reacting to was the lack of connection, feeling of being controlled, and not being seen, heard, or understood.

Connection, Not Coercion

Where does connection come from?

Connection comes from two main places: joy and vulnerability. Connection through joy usually looks like shared experiences, heightened positive emotions, and love. Most parents simply expect this to come easily since, after all, you gave birth to your child and the relationship should automatically default to joy, which leads to connection, right? But that isn't always the case, and we'll be exploring more on this belief throughout the book.

"When you keep criticizing your kids, they don't stop loving you. They stop loving themselves. Let that sink in."
~ Author Unknown

Second, connection comes from vulnerability. Vulnerability breeds connection. As a parent, you must also be transparent with your adolescent and be willing to share your own struggles, unresolved traumas, and the beliefs you've held tightly as a vaulted part of your identity. In order to help connect with your teens, you need to be willing to look at your blind spots, which appear as unquestioned beliefs based on your own upbringing or life experiences. You must be willing to face your fears and unpack what beliefs you've formed about yourself.

How do we know the fears are there? Feel your way through this; you will know.

Your teens know your fears too because they are keyed into which buttons to push. Right?

Just notice every time you are triggered and pull the authority card. You will know when you expect your teen's behavior to match your expectations of them. You will know when you take things personally, when you perceive

77

your teen's behavior as rude, when they make "stupid" mistakes, when they push your buttons, and when they embarrass you.

One of the best tools I discovered on my own parenting journey was to stop, consider, and internally inquire, "Does this statement, reaction, or comment I am about to make promote connection, or is it designed to coerce?" I'll admit, this takes tremendous commitment, requiring practice and ultimately failure. However, when you have the deep desire to live in partnership, this question becomes as natural as breathing.

Trust me, as parents, we recognize many situations that have that effect on us. And to be clear, this is not only our teen's work; this is our work too. If we allow these moments of judgment, expectations, embarrassment, or disappointment to become our dominant experience with our teens, we are not connecting. For the tools found within this book to have any impact, you must choose connection over coercion at all costs.

Yes, you have your work to do as a parent too.

Finally, cultivate a practice of being truly present. It takes commitment and patience to be present in your own life, let alone in the life of someone else. Recognize when you prioritize your to-do list, your schedule, and your responsibilities over noticing the light in your teen's eyes, how they may be feeling, what beautiful things have changed in them, and where the small openings for connection lie.

In modern life, we often don't have time and tend to overlook these small things. You could be missing the opportunity. This is your permission to put down your phone, do the dishes later, stop whatever you are doing, and simply observe and be present. These moments do not arise often in the teen universe, and they are easily missed. Your teen might not have the words but truly has the desire to feel connected. You might have missed their silent invitation. Becoming present, willing, and accountable takes some practice. When the parent is not present or available, the teen responds in kind. If you are noticing negative and destructive cycles in your teen, please honestly look at your willingness to be unconditionally present for them.

What does it mean to be present? The present parent is available and lets their teen know they are there for them. They are open to discussing anything, without judgment or control. The present parent can offer advice or solutions but not be attached to their teen following it. The present parent doesn't judge their teen's mistakes and helps their teen unpack the natural consequences of their actions. The present parent helps their teen set healthy limits around their body and safety. The present parent is available but never controlling. The present parent is never dismissive and acts with kindness, always trying to bring levity to the most stressful situations. The present parent shows up for their teen without conditions.

Attachment Parenting

The way we are connected is often referred to as "attachment." Attachment Parenting focuses on nurturing connection between a parent and a child. Most Attachment Parenting literature, research, and philosophy address early childhood development. There is much science-backed literature correlating parenting styles to brain development, concluding that healthy parent-child relationships that embody empathy, responsiveness, and love-oriented parenting produce securely attached adults.

According to API (Attachment Parenting International):

> Attachment Parenting is an approach to childrearing that promotes a secure attachment bond between parents and their children. Attachment is a scientific term for the emotional bond in a relationship. The attachment quality that forms between parents and children, learned from the relational patterns with caregivers from birth on, correlates with how a child perceives – and ultimately is able to experience – relationships. Attachment quality is correlated with lifelong effects and often much more profound an impact than people understand. A person with a secure attachment is generally able to respond to stress in healthy ways and establish more meaningful and close relationships more often; a person with an insecure attachment style may be more susceptible to stress and less

healthy relationships. A greater number of insecurely attached individuals are at risk for more serious mental health concerns such as depression and anxiety.

From a parenting perspective, our goal is to connect with our children by meeting their needs for trust, empathy, and affection by providing consistent, loving, and responsive care. That's easier said than done, of course. Many of us do that naturally, especially in our child's younger years, but when our children reach adolescence, everything is out the window. Admittedly, it's much easier to maintain an attached relationship if we've practiced the philosophy with our teen since birth, but in case you didn't, you can start from this point forward, embodying the information in this book.

If you aren't familiar with Attachment Parenting, I urge you to dig in. There is a robust reference section in the Suggested Reading section and within Chapter 5, we will unpack attachment theory.

Before Miro was born, I started reading about the philosophy and the psychology behind Attachment Parenting. I discovered my insecure attachment style was known as disorganized attachment, which is one of the three types of insecure attachments. This led me down a path of personal healing so I could raise Miro with a secure attachment, in order to best prepare him for life. I found the principles of Attachment Parenting useful and although most literature is written for parents of younger children, I continued to practice Attachment Parenting throughout his adolescence and beyond.

Here are the eight principles of Attachment Parenting I've adapted specifically for parenting teens:

1. Prepare for Parenting a Teen: The overarching message within this principle is the importance of parents healing their own attachment wounds, taking responsibility for their own triggers, and being accountable and transparent in their relationships within family.
2. Act with Love, Respect, and Kindness: Kindness goes a long way. Oftentimes, we can be tempted to counter our teen's aloof behavior with an equal or more severe reaction. It's our work not to take their

behavior personally and watch our own triggers and expectations. They express exactly how they are feeling and that takes trust. Recognize that it isn't about you and respond with kindness and love.

3. Respond with Sensitivity: This principle is a central element of all the principles, and it is viewed by many parents as the cornerstone of Attachment Parenting. It encompasses a timely response by a nurturing caregiver. You need to hone your skills to determine what your teen needs. Do they really need to be trusted with time and space to work things out? Or are they craving someone to listen to them without trying to solve their problems or judge their experience?

4. Be Nurturing: Infants require nurturing touch to feel they are safe and cared for. Teens, however, speak a totally different language. Discover your teen's Love Language and explore if and how they respond to acts of kindness, touch, words, or time spent together. Honor their style and provide nurturing in the language they speak.

5. Encourage Teens to Listen to Their Bodies: Our bodies are designed to function perfectly, but during adolescence, it's really a time of change. Support your teens to really know what is working for their bodies and what is no longer working. Encourage your teens to get deep rest when they are tired, eat when they are hungry, and move or exercise daily.

6. Use Consistent and Loving Care: Secure attachment depends on continuity of care. Become that rock your teen needs and assure them you are available and present.

7. Guide By Values, Not Rules: Connection is fractured through punitive discipline techniques. Instead, connect through values and become the guidepost as your teen develops his or her own sense of moral responsibility within the construct of the family value system and the greater world.

8. Strive for Personal and Family Balance: Attachment Parenting is a family-centered approach in which all members of the family have equal value. The parent is not a tyrant, yet also not a martyr. Parents need to balance their parenting role and their personal life in order to continue having the energy and motivation to maintain a healthy relationship and to model healthy lifestyles for their children.

Partnering With Your Teen

In addition to the principles of Attachment Parenting, I urge you to consider parenting in partnership with your teens. In Chapter 2, I introduced and defined partnership parenting and the partnership parenting paradigm. Here, I will share some specifics and attempt to provide a deeper understanding of how to apply these strategies to your own parenting. So, let's dig in...

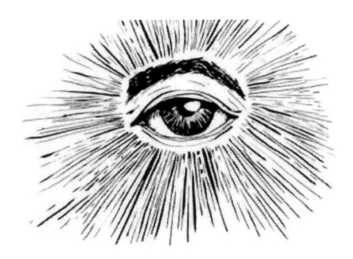

If you're serious about change, you have to go through uncomfortable situations. Stop trying to dodge the process. It's the only way to grow.

Challenging Authority

Just to be clear, authoritarian parenting is the opposite of partnership parenting. When you are in partnership, no single person has authority over another person. But isn't it true you, as the parent, are legally, financially, and culturally responsible for your teens? Of course. Within all partnerships, different parties maintain different roles and responsibilities.

Think of the task of creating a website. You may be working with a creative designer, a talented writer, a resourceful coder, and even an organized project manager. All members of the team are moving towards a single goal together, each bringing with them a unique set of talents and approaches. There will be times when each member of the team takes the lead and shares a different perspective in the case of problem-solving. And in a perfect world, no one member is more important than another. Ideally, each member must work together, keeping the end goal in mind. They do so by remaining in communication, being respectful of others' points of view, being accountable and responsible for their daily tasks, and adjusting as needed.

Granted, raising a teen is nothing like designing a website (I've done both), and we all know within that scenario, the client is ultimately the boss. What we can take from that example is the desire to work creatively together, practice deep communication, learn to see things from different perspectives, collaborate, employ compromise when necessary, and focus on the goal at hand.

In the professional world, when things go wrong, mistakes are made, or deadlines are missed, there are natural consequences. In some cases, the team may have to do the project over, be forced to make concessions, work extra hours, or ultimately lose the project or even their job. You will never find a situation where the coder demands the designer doesn't design for 3 weeks or the project manager is forbidden to turn their computer on for a week as punishment.

Even though the analogy above is flawed and raising teens is nothing like designing a website, what we can take from this story is that each contributor to the project brings a different and unique point of view or talent. You, as the parent, have years of experience, you take on the roles you take on in the family, and your teens are exactly where they should be in terms of their talents, experiences, and perspectives.

In parenting a teen, there is no end goal. Sure, we want our teens to grow into joyful adults, but the only way they can do that is by having a clear "present goal." You must bring your present goal to the partnership to make sure your teen is always seen, heard, and understood.

Understand that partnerships are not always equal, nor is the responsibility of parenting. You have a lot on your shoulders in general, and within the partnership paradigm, there will always be an ebb and a flow, frustrations, and joys. But keep in mind, the key to all relationships is communication, kindness, and grace. Don't commit to being in partnership within a vacuum. Please share with your teen what partnership means to you and ask them what it means to them. Invite your teen to be an active partner with you and to help keep you accountable to your commitments. Promise you won't get angry when they are pointing out when you are being authoritative, let them know you are working on your internal world too, and it's a process and a journey you wish to share with them.

Demanding your teen to do something because you have authority over them because you "said so" or because you are responsible for them is the antithesis of being in a partnership paradigm.

What does it mean to be in partnership? All parties need to choose to be in partnership. Sit down with your teen, let them know you wish to try parenting in this approach, and ask them what partnership means to them. Ask them what roles, talents, perspectives, and skills they bring to the partnership. Discuss what responsibility each member of the partnership should bring and how each member of the partnership can help support one another. Finally, practice communication. Practice again and again. It's called practice because it's never perfected, never completed, and always changing and nuanced.

I share some suggestions in the final chapter, so when you are finished reading this book, you will be ready to get started.

Parenting Without Rules

What? How can we even consider life without rules, let alone parenting a teen? Doesn't that guarantee complete chaos in the home, out-of-control teens, lack of responsibility, and dangerous situations?

Absolutely not. I'm going to share with you how in just a moment.
We just explored the nature of authoritarian parenting. Commonly, authoritarian parents create rules, oftentimes many of them. This requires the parents to be the rule-makers, the rule-enforcer, and if the rules are broken, the rule-punisher. Most rules made in families are based on two things: the convenience of the parent and the desire to control the teen's behavior. Neither of these goals promotes connection, and they tend to damage relationships. Furthermore, rules are generally arbitrary by nature. Why must a teen be in bed by 10:00 pm? Why not at 10:22 pm? My response would be, why should there be any rules around bedtimes, food, activity, behavior, or performance anyway? Don't natural consequences occur? Doesn't the experience of those consequences provide information about the best choices to make?

This kind of living requires a highly engaged parent, who can provide information, help teens see potential consequences, and help them discover the effect their choices can have on their lives. This kind of living requires a parent who can support their teen to make mistakes in a safe space, unpack the consequences, explore safety and the nature of well-being, and do so without judgment of any kind. Learning from this kind of engagement is deep, and the intrinsic motivation to make choices for oneself based on natural consequences helps young people define their own morals and values.

"If children feel safe, they can take risks, ask questions, make mistakes, learn to trust, share their feelings, and grow."
~ Alfie Kohn

Many of us grew up in households where we heard the words, "If you are going to live in my house, you must live by my rules!" That's the way it was, and most of us just accepted this is the way the world operates. Many adults raised under those conditions believe living by rules taught them morals and how to function in society. I've heard this statement from many of the parents I've worked with, and their conditioning runs deep. Although it's true that they may have learned morals and values, they were morals and values that came from someone else versus from within. Morals and values adapted from an authoritarian source are not really a person's own morals and values. They are conditioning and, in some cases, indoctrination. The richness of raising individuals is the opportunity to discover and find your own moral compass and the core values that bring meaning to your own life.

In fact, core values are at the heart of living a life without rules. In Chapter 9, I provide a powerful tool for discovering the core values you are currently living and defining the core values you aspire to adapt. Imagine a family that knows their core values. Each individual knows what's important to them, and the direction of their moral compass is understood. Now imagine a family who has taken the time to define the values they share as a family. Now imagine a challenge or decision that needs to be made. The question simply remains, "Is this choice in alignment with my/the family's core values?" This is the key to defining your true north. No rules necessary. And eventually, this is the key to raising a self-actualized, morally driven adult, which is exactly what the world truly needs.

Rewards & Punishment

"If I offered you a thousand dollars to take off your shoes, you'd very likely accept--and then I could triumphantly announce that 'rewards work.' But as with punishments, they can never help someone develop a *commitment* to a task or action, a reason to keep doing it when there's no longer a payoff."
~ Alfie Kohn

It's likely obvious at this point that a rewards and punishment model is not comparable with partnership parenting. This approach turns homes into battlefields, encouraging a win-or-lose environment. As you can imagine, this approach kills connection and threatens to transform parents into lazy, disconnected, unconscious parents. Think about it, it takes much less effort to live in a black-or-white rule-based home than to be in dialogue with your teen about all the gray spaces in between.

Second, let's consider years of consistent and compelling scientific research examining if the rewards and punishment model is effective.

In Alfie Kohn's book, *Unconditional Parenting: Moving from Rewards and Punishments to Love and Reason,* Kohn unpacks the psychology of living in a punitive environment from the child's perspective. If the child (or in our case, the adolescent) perceives the role of their parents as someone who will punish them and ultimately make them suffer, they are not developing a loving connection. Defenders of conventional parenting argue this mean-spirited approach is for the child's own good. Yet, studies show the complete opposite is true.

Kohn reports on these studies in his book. He references a classic parenting study involving younger children and their mothers from the 1950s in which researchers found that "the unhappy effects of punishment have run like a dismal thread through our findings" and consistently found that punishment was "ineffectual over the long term as a technique for eliminating the kind of behavior toward which it is directed."

In his book, he also cites more recent and well-designed studies which serve to strengthen this conclusion, finding, for example, that parents who practice punishing rule-breaking behavior at home often have children who demonstrate higher levels of rule-breaking when they are away from the home.

Barbara Coloroso, author of *Kids Are Worth It!: Giving Your Child the Gift of Inner Discipline,* says parents of teenagers often say, "He was such a good kid, so well behaved, so well mannered, so well dressed. Now look at him!" She offers the following reply, "From the time he was young, he dressed the way you told him to dress; he acted the way you told him to act; he said the things you told him to say. He's been listening to somebody else tell him what to do…he hasn't changed."

Experiencing autonomy is vitally important during this stage. If we choose to parent our teens through control, punishments and rewards, and rules instead of values, we are affecting their development. Remember, your adolescent's brain is in the middle of a profound process of remodeling, and their sense of identity is unfolding each and every day. Consider the long-term impact controlling behavior may have on them. Are you setting them up to normalize being controlled by others? Consider how this may play out in their adult relationships with their future peers and partners.

Seeing Our Teens for Who They Are *Right Now*

As parents, we often see our children through the cumulative lens and through the things they've recently done, which may be an indication of the development phase they are in. We often view them as the ones who didn't pick up their clothes, overslept, or left dirty dishes in the sink. In reality, none of that is important. What is stopping them from blossoming into who they are becoming is us, as parents, who are guilty of seeing them through our cumulative reduction. Partnering with them is about showing up for them and being who they need in this exact moment, not parenting a past version of your child.

How do we partner?
- Recognize and honor they are becoming more independent.
- Create space for them to make decisions and let them know you trust them.
- Support their mistakes. You cannot jump in and tell them not to do things or beat them up for doing it and failing.
- Help them unpack all of the unseen consequences.

Your own adolescence experience is very different from your teen's, and depending on where you are in your healing process, it is important not to expect your teen to be in the same place. Partnering with your own inner-teen is going to give you the cues and clues on how to support your adolescent. What did you need as a teen and didn't get? Were you supported? Did anyone encourage you to step out of your comfort zone? Were you living in the present? Did you miss out on something because you weren't? How does this inform your teen's expectation of what life should be like?

After taking a step back to look at things in this light, you may find out you are parenting a totally different teen than the image of your teen you've created in your mind. The fulfilled, safe, and secure inner-teen will allow you to exhale and be the partner your actual teen needs. This entire book is about self-inquiry and not projecting your story or baggage onto your teen. The thought process of "I am going to make sure you don't make the same mistakes I did" may be coming from a place of concern, but there is judgment about one's self that is unresolved, and it turns into automatic judgment about your teen's actions.

Fear & Internal Monologues

We are all human. There are thousands of conversations happening in our heads at all times whether we are aware of them or not. From deciding what to have for dinner, why the driver cuts you off on the way to work, or what you are doing for the weekend. Those are the routine, mundane monologues.

Oftentimes, they are related to agendas. These agendas are like a glorified laundry list of the expected outcomes from a non-consenting third party, such as your teen. These conversations and agendas are happening because of our own fears surrounding a particular outcome. Some of these monologues might sound like this:
- He's so lazy.
- She will never graduate.
- They are going to live at home forever.

As parents, we need to keep this in check and not let it influence how we interact with our children. They are likely not sharing in the same fear-driven thoughts about their potential future and projecting our own generational wounds and fears onto them is not going to inspire them to reach their full potential.

So how do we parent and partner without these agendas? The key is to uncover two things: 1.) the expectation of experiencing a particular thing in a particular way and 2.) fears that lie just below our thoughts. Ultimately, you may find as you explore your own mind that these two things are linked to each other.

Some thoughts are conscious like, "I want what's best for my teen." That is what most parents want of course. The agenda you may uncover is the expectation of what exactly that may look like. Of course, we tend to default back to, "But I only want what's best for them," but what we are really doing in our minds is creating the correct or appropriate path as a result of that thought. Furthermore, we weave our fears into the mix with secretive thoughts like, "If they don't achieve _____ by this time, they will _____." (Example: If they don't achieve good study habits by the time they are 15, they will never find a job and live in my basement until they are 37).

Take a moment of deep self-inquiry now. Grab a notebook or use the blank pages at the end of this book to write out what your private fear is. Commit it to paper and recognize what fears you've been holding on to.

Once you've defined your thought, ask yourself, how long have you been practicing this thought? Have you been habitually thinking this thought so often it's become a belief? Is this thought connected to the emotion of fear? Notice what other emotions are attached to the fear when you are consciously thinking the thoughts.

Now, think of all the ways this thought, fear, and belief have influenced your interactions with your teen. List them out now.

Most of the time, we have buried this thought/fear/belief so deeply with shame that we don't share it with others, let alone ourselves. But bringing this private, sometimes secret, fear or belief to the forefront of our conscious mind makes it easier to look at it, analyze it, and even challenge it. These thoughts, fears, and beliefs can creep into all our interactions, not only with our teens but within all of our relationships. As much as we think we are keeping these things hidden, I've got news for you, your kids know they are there. They may not know the exact contents of your particular thought/fear/belief, but they sense it in the form of an agenda.

This is our work within the partnership. This is deep work.

Triggers & Accountability

WHAT {TRIGGERED} ME

1. I felt excluded.
2. I felt powerless.
3. I felt unheard.
4. I felt scolded.
5. I felt jugged.
6. I felt blamed.
7. I felt disrespected.
8. I felt a lack of affection.
9. I felt I couldn't speak up.
10. I felt unseen.
11. I felt ignored.
12. I felt I couldn't be honest.
13. I felt like the bad guy.
14. I felt forgotten.
15. I felt unsafe.
16. I felt unloved.
17. I felt like it was unfair.
18. I felt frustrated.
19. I felt disconnected.
20. I felt trapped.
21. I felt a lack of passion.
22. I felt uncared for.
23. I felt manipulated.
24. I felt controlled.

When we speak about triggers, most parents immediately start to rattle off all the things that "trigger" their teen. Whether it's asking them to do their chores, communicate about their day, or simply respond when spoken to, the adult brain thinks we have triggered the response from the teen. But in this section, we are going to focus on the triggers of the parent.

In partnership parenting or working with a teen on any level, any unresolved trauma the parent has endured in their own life will surface and play into the relationship as much, or more than, the teen trauma. We are going to cover this in much more detail in Chapter 6 but understanding the concept as it relates to triggers and accountability is worth mentioning here. As adults, we don't always look back at our past and work to identify what may have hurt us. Oftentimes, we bury our traumas in order to cope with everyday life as part of our natural survival instinct. This works as a short-term strategy, but eventually, something is going to bring it straight to the surface.

When a teen first comes home and walks right past you without saying hello, it could trigger a reaction based on the expectation (realistic or not) that they should have been pleasant. This triggers the parent to feel dismissed, possibly as they did in their own younger years. A parent may approach their teen demanding a response but may be subconsciously seeking a resolution to their own childhood wounds. Because parents are in an artificial position of authority, they may try to assert the control they did not have in their own childhood.

The expectation of the parent that triggers their emotional response is not the same as the expectation of the teen who does not think they did anything wrong. Because of this disconnect, the result is most commonly an overreaction on the part of the parent, not the teen. The first step in fixing this is to learn how to separate the expectation from the trigger. The second step is recognizing when you, as the parent, are having this emotional response to the trigger that stems from a belief system that is yours and not the teen's.

Your trigger is your work and no one else's. The act of being triggered is brought to light as conscious or more likely unconscious beliefs are challenged and old wounds are activated. One of the best ways to accomplish this is to work on self-inquiry, a concept we will discuss in more detail at the end of this chapter.

Even after becoming efficient in self-inquiry, recognize it is not your teen's responsibility to stop everything going on in their brain so they can accommodate your beliefs. Teens are experiencing their own triggers too, but yours are likely more profoundly layered.

On the opposite side of the coin, teen triggers (whatever it is that sets them off) are not the problem of the parent. The parent needs to focus on themselves and let the teen focus on what they are going through. In the 13-16 age range, a lot of the triggers teens experience are somehow rooted in how parents are pushing them to start looking inward and become more independent. Teens want more space, and a parent's natural response is to give them less space.

A young man I'm working with, when asked the percentage of time he feels like his mom is "on his team," told me it was less than 50%. He explained to me that his mother expects him to do chores he doesn't think he should be responsible for, and she often confronts him to talk about things he's not comfortable talking about with her. He viewed this as a deliberate attempt to stop him from self-actualizing so she could push her own agenda on him, which in turn triggered him to believe there was a lack of connection between them, thus on opposite teams. This is perceived very differently from the teen's perspective than from the parent's perspective. The parent is being triggered because of their own traumas, and in turn, it is creating new traumas in their adolescent. It is the beginning of a vicious cycle.

When the teen feels forced to connect, it is the antithesis of connection. Their default belief is that the parent is controlling. Knowing this, the accountability component is the responsibility of the parent. As a parent learns to be accountable and reach for connection instead of coercion, they must make efforts to repair. Repair looks like this:

- Being aware of and identifying your own triggers.
- Sharing those triggers with family members so there is awareness and transparency. One of the best ways to create connection is

through vulnerability. It also shows there is fallibility in being human and having shit to deal with. There's nothing wrong with having it, but how you deal with it matters, and sharing that can allow the other person to hold us accountable for ourselves.

- Continually working on our triggers.
- Recognizing the difference between reaction and response.
- Being aware of the impact the reaction/response has on the connection and relationship.

I realized the importance of everything we just covered through specific interactions with my own child. When Miro would tell me I was acting like my mother, it would shut me down and cause me to be more reflective because this is the absolute worst thing he could ever say to me. I have done so much work to heal those traumas, but there are still moments when they get the best of me. It can be hard to realize that as people we will never be done working on ourselves. This has much to do with our relationship with ourselves as well as our relationships with our teens and others that might trigger us.

I invite you to consider the nature of relationships and how they are a powerful tool for healing yourself and healing your family. In fact, you cannot heal your patterns, triggers, or traumas without being in "relationship" with others. It's true that all healing is an inside job, but that's only half of the story. The other half is to be in relationships with others as your healed self in order to reprogram the neural pathways or integrate the stuff you are healing into a new way of being. You can only do this in relationships with other people. I'll repeat this, there is no way to heal your childhood or ancestral wounds in a vacuum. You must be in relationships with other people, and your teen, who is doing a great job triggering you and making you look at this stuff, is the perfect person to heal with. How's that for partnership?

Because triggers play such a vital role in how we relate to our teens, being what they are and how they make us feel, it is paramount to keep track of when they happen and what our response is. The trigger can be a person, place, or thing that evokes a certain emotion or response from us of varying intensity. For that reason, I have created the trigger log below to help both parents and teens become more aware of what happens, when, and how we react to it. Commit to logging your own triggers, starting now, for one full week.

Date & Time	Trigger (What happened?)	Level of Intensity (1-10)	Emotion(s) (What did you feel?)	Response (What did you do?)

Strategies When Triggered

First thing's first: What exactly is a trigger?

A trigger is anything that causes your brain to believe you are experiencing a threat, even if you are perfectly safe. We become triggered because we've encountered something, usually sensory, that consciously or subconsciously reminds us of a particular negative event from our past. This can be that thought we've been habitually thinking, which has transformed into a belief, or it can be a past trauma.

Dr. Aimee Daramus, author of *The Stress Switch: The Truth About Stress and How to Short-Circuit,* says encountering a trigger can cause our bodies to go into fight, flight, or freeze mode as if we're experiencing a past trauma at that moment.

"There's a big reduction in activity in the 'thinking' parts of the brain, which help you with planning, organizing and impulse control," Daramus explains. "There's a lot of activity in the survival parts of the brain, including the centers for fear and aggression. So you're scared, upset [and] feeling as if there's an emergency even if there isn't. And your brain is scared, ready to defend itself, and not thinking as clearly as usual."

When you find yourself in flight, flight, or freeze mode while parenting, your teen may be transformed into your nemesis (in your mind). In addition to the emotional reaction, you will experience the biological effects including hormones and neurotransmitters flooding your body, causing your muscles to tense, your pulse to race, and your breathing to quicken. Notice how that feels in your body, which response is dominant, and in which order it occurs. In all reality, when you are in a triggered state, it's not going to be easy to parent in partnership.

Here are 10 suggestions to follow when you are triggered by your teen:

1. **Commit to noticing when you are getting triggered.**

   By using the trigger log, you are training your conscious mind to recognize when you are being triggered. You may notice the signs through the situation, the welling up of emotions, or even the thoughts coming up. Take time to notice the biological changes in your body as well. Become the expert on your own triggers, learn to focus attention inward when it starts, and wire your subconscious mind to alert your conscious mind as a sort of early warning system.

2. **Don't take action when you are triggered.**

   When triggered, remember these three words: stop, drop (your agenda), and breathe. Remember, taking a deep breath can be as powerful as pushing a pause button. Pausing gives you options, allowing you to choose a response instead of auto-reacting. Consciously choose to breathe over speaking. Notice what feelings are inhabiting your body. Recognize them, give them names, and notice if one emotion is dominant and actually covering up other emotions. Often, anger masks fear, sadness, or disappointment. Breathe into the feelings and honor that they are there.

3.   **Take five.**

Recognize that when you are triggered, it is a terrible starting place to talk it out. Instead, give yourself time away and come back when you're able to be calm. Honor your teen by honestly letting them know your state, by saying something like, "I need a few minutes. I'm too upset/angry/enraged to be rational right now. I'll be back soon." Use this time to calm yourself and do not work yourself into a deeper frenzy. Sometimes running your hands under cold water and focusing on the feelings you are experiencing helps. Just make sure you don't get into a thought loop, justifying just how "right" you are. When you have calmed, return.

4.   **Listen, watch, and observe your thoughts and feelings.**

Remember our exploration into emotions when we discussed the Trauma Train in Chapter 2? Flip back and review now, if you have to. Those lessons apply to us here too. If you are feeling anger, sit with it, understand all the emotions wrapped up in it, and unpack what information it's giving you. If you can, uncover the thoughts or beliefs it's tied to as well. You'll benefit from this exercise. These emotions are a great source of information on the road to healing our own traumas.

5.   **Don't act until you've completely cooled down.**

Recognize that acting on your anger oftentimes reinforces and escalates it. Despite the popular belief that we need to express our anger to get it out, recognize there is nothing constructive about expressing anger *at* another person, especially your teen. Research shows expressing anger while we are angry makes us angrier. Sounds like a toxic cycle you might want to avoid.

6. **Always avoid physical force.**

An alarming 85% of adolescents say they've been slapped or spanked by their parents (Journal of Psychopathology, 2007). There are numerous studies proving physical punishment has a negative impact on children's development that lasts throughout their lives. As you can imagine, physical force ultimately sabotages connection, fractures your relationship, and thrusts you into an authoritarian model of parenting. Do everything you can to not apply force, and if you can't control yourself, get some help.

7. **Avoid threats.**

Threats are absolutely not in alignment with partnership parenting. If you make a threat while you are triggered, they will likely be irrational, unreasonable, and maybe even hurtful. Since threats ultimately require the person making them follow through, they place you outside of the partnership paradigm and ultimately undermine your connection and relationship. Instead, after you've calmed, help your teen unpack the natural consequences of their choices and shift your stance to being there to assist them to face whatever is next.

8. **Be aware of your tone and word choice.**

This is a tricky and personal tip depending on you, your family culture, and your tendencies. I can say the nicest words, but if there is a hint of aggression in there, Miro will know instantly and call me out as being passive-aggressive. However, research shows that the more calmly we speak, the calmer we feel and the more calmly others respond to us. I would not suggest acting calm; however, I'd suggest showing up authentically calm. Use the power to calm yourself and invite your teen to match your mood.

9. **Choose your battles.**

Early in my adult relationships, I noticed I had the impulse to prove how "right" I was. This was because I wasn't heard in my childhood and adolescence. As I started to heal these wounds, I was able to select what was important to me to fight over and what was not worth it. If your teen does something that drives you crazy like leaving their shoes in the living room, isn't that more about you than your teen? It may not be worth it to pursue and instead recognize it's really your work.

10. **Acknowledge that you are part of the problem.**

If you're open to emotional growth, your teen will always show you where you need to focus. If you're not, it's impossible to be a partnership parent because you'll always get triggered and potentially be your worst. Take responsibility to manage your own emotional well-being first. Your teen may not become an angel overnight, but you'll be amazed to see how much less disconnected they are once you model taking responsibility for your own mental health.

Fixing Your Teen's Behavior

We've already shown that punishment and rewards are not effective ways of parenting. However, most parents, who think punishment and rewards are an effective way to parent, are really trying to control one thing: their teen's behavior.

Dr. Shefali Tsabury, the author of *The Conscious Parent*, describes this kind of parenting as a "prisoner-warden" approach. The "warden-parent" must closely monitor the "prisoner-teen's" behaviors and determine if they are either "right" or "wrong." The "warden-parent" then must prescribe the appropriate punishment or reward. However, the unforeseen result of this type of engagement is that the "prisoner-teen" becomes dependent on the "warden-parent" to regulate their behavior. I write more about the nature of self-regulation in Chapter 6.

"It's because discipline focuses on behavior, not on the feelings driving the behavior, that it undercuts the very thing we are trying to accomplish."
~ Dr. Shefali Tsabury

Discipline is a tricky topic. Many of us developed a relationship with that word in our own childhoods. Some feel it's a good thing, others do not. When discipline is applied by an authority to a child, it is not in alignment with the principles in this book. However, I have developed a beautiful relationship with the word discipline by adding the word "self" before it. Learning self-discipline isn't a bad thing.

My final note on this topic: I suspect there may have been a reader or two who picked up this book with hopes of learning how to modify their teen's behavior. I suspect they've also put this book down by now. To be clear, there will never be any hint of a suggestion on how to manipulate your teen into behaving differently. This is just not in alignment with partnership parenting.

Learning How to Repair

Growing up, I never heard my mother say to me the words, "I'm sorry," unless it was in the context of "I'm sorry, but NO!" As a child, apologies were something I was expected to do a lot until one day my mother said, "Don't apologize if you don't mean it!" I remember the feeling of power welling up in my little body as I replied with a defiant one-word response, "OK!"

Apologies, in my childhood and adolescence experience, had never felt like a repair. Instead, they were my obligation and were merely a tool to appease.

Internally, there was a lot happening in my subconscious landscape. Apologies were the messenger to my brain that I was defective and faulty. They underscored the belief I already had about myself, "I am not enough."

Throughout my life, I've had a hard time believing when others apologized to me that they could possibly be authentic in meaning. After all, how could I be worthy of receiving an apology if I wasn't actually "enough"?

In my youth, the ruptures between my primary caretaker (my mother) and myself were never repaired. When ruptures occurred, I had to self-soothe, finding safety in my private tears under the covers of my bed or locked in the bathroom. Adolescence was especially hard for me after I recognized no repairs would be made. I had to be reliant on myself.

During adolescence, I remember craving to be seen, heard, and understood from the depths of my soul, dreaming of a mother who opened my bedroom door at night, sat gently on the edge of my bed, and softly apologized for not being kind to me. I craved to hear the words, "I'm so sorry, Lainie," as she stroked my hair and wiped away my salty tears. Those experiences never happened, words never came nor were repairs ever made, and all the thoughts about my waning self-worth compounded deeper into my subconscious mind.

A developing brain can translate many of our early childhood experiences into shadow beliefs about ourselves. We touch on this in Chapter 5 Without having our caretakers take time to repair ruptures when they happen, the trauma can cut deep.

I can tell you our teens want and need the reassurance that comes from repair. Being right is never more important than the connection of the relationship. The situations ebb and flow, and mistakes are made as life moves on, but the opportunities to repair ruptures, fights, and disagreements through kindness and compassion heal like no other elixir.

For parents, our egos may get in the way. But heartfelt apologies are greater than the situation itself, fault, the act of being right (or wrong), or teaching them a lesson. Parents who model how to repair a rupture with their teens help them understand accountability, our human fallibility, and the value of connection.

Remember, there is no such thing as the perfect way of behaving in a relationship. Relationships require vulnerability, and you must give yourself the time and permission to be reflective about the role you played in the rupture. Be honest with yourself. Then, you must have enough trust in yourself to objectively verbalize your reflections and take responsibility for your words and actions with your teen. "I was wrong" or "I made a mistake" are very powerful words. It requires compassion to apologize from the heart and hold yourself accountable. The same holds true for making a reconnection. Maintain open lines of communication, especially when the inevitable ruptures in connection occur. Our own deep understanding of ourselves, our past traumas, our triggers, and our shortcomings are essential because our buttons will inevitably be pushed. As your adolescent goes through changes. I promise you'll have plenty of opportunities to practice repair on this journey. Have fun with it!

Self-Inquiry

I've mentioned self-inquiry countless times in this book already, but I think it's prudent to dedicate an entire section to this. Self-inquiry is the simplest action of looking at your own self and questioning, exploring, examining, or investigating ANYTHING regarding oneself.

> SELF: Refers to a person or individual.
> INQUIRY: Means investigation, examination, exploration, question.

Self-inquiry can be thought of as a kind of mindfulness practice in which you ask yourself good or probing questions. One of the desired outcomes of practicing self-inquiry is to dive deep into your mind to help you find your personal unknown. By exploring those spaces, sometimes found in our deep unconscious, we are seeking to understand our experiences in new ways, thus allowing ourselves to develop new behaviors and change old patterns.

As we practice self-inquiry, we are seeking the spaces in our minds, which are oftentimes filled with discomfort. These are the spaces we hold our struggles, beliefs, criticisms, and fears. Much of the time, we'll notice each of those beliefs is anchored in emotion, and sometimes it feels like we are pulling out a never-ending clown's handkerchief. We can often feel self-inquiry in our bodies through the tightness in the chest, rapid breathing, butterflies in the stomach, clenching fists, numbness, and the desire to walk away. If you are experiencing those physical symptoms, you are there.

Here are some things to keep in mind as you commit to practicing self-inquiry:

- Self-inquiry involves a willingness to courageously challenge our beliefs, convictions, and perceptions of what we identify as the "truth."
- Self-inquiry acknowledges that we don't see the world as it is, rather we see the world as we are.
- Self-inquiry is uncomfortable and sometimes difficult.
- Self-inquiry recognizes every new understanding is limited, fallible, and potentially biased.
- Self-inquiry requires taking responsibility for our beliefs, choices, and perceptions rather than blaming others.
- Self-inquiry requires practice and patience.
- You must commit to not judging yourself through the self-inquiry process.

Self-inquiry can be practiced in many ways, through journaling, meditation, and simple reflection. It can also be used in conjunction with another framework. A simple example of a framework is considering the introvert/extrovert framework. Look at these simplified definitions of both:

> **Introvert:** a person whose personality is characterized by introversion: a typically reserved or quiet person who tends to be introspective and enjoys spending time alone
> **Extrovert:** a person whose personality is characterized by extroversion: a typically gregarious and unreserved person who enjoys and seeks out social interaction

Your selection or identification with either introvert or extrovert is not important here, but you could not access an external source for the answer. Instead, you must check inside and ask yourself, "Which am I?" You can do the same with any other external framework like horoscopes, Love Languages, Myers-Briggs personality tests, or any number of countless other examples.

Through self-inquiry, we can access many layers within ourselves. Some are easily accessible while others we have to dig deep for. The questions we ask are the key, and many of the tools we use in Chapter 9 will invite you to look below the surface.

I'm going to get you started now with a self-inquiry challenge. I urge you to do this challenge yourself first, think about it deeply and reflect. Afterwards, ask your teen to do the same challenge. The reason is two-fold. First, you may discover something about yourself you've never considered or articulated. Second, you may discover what your teen actually wants and needs.

Challenge

Consider your innermost truth. Ask yourself, what do you want or need in your life right **NOW** to satisfy your innermost desires?

On the left-hand side, rate its importance in your life using a scale of 1 to 10, 1 being the least important and 10 being the most. In the second column, rate from 1 to 10 what you are living or experiencing now in your current circumstance. Be honest.

Importance in My Life 1-10	Currently Living 1-10	Quality	Description
		Certainty & Security	*Control of situations, consistency, routine, safety*
		Variety & Spontaneity	*Surprises, challenges, adventures, unpredictability*
		Significance	*Need to feel important & valued, noticed for who you are, recognized & valued for accomplishments, acknowledged*
		Connection & Love	*Intimacy, feeling part of something, bonding, touch*
		Growth	*Expand knowledge, comfort zones, relationships*
		Contribution	*Desire to give, share, provide, feel unity & make a difference*
		Freedom & Independence	*Independent, untethered, self-governing, sovereign*

Unpacking the challenge

How do you feel after completing this exercise? Did you discover anything about what you desire and what you are currently living? Did any feelings or beliefs come up? Did you experience a "should" thought that conflicted with what you truly wanted? If there was conflict, did it bring up any emotions? Can you find some beliefs hidden below those emotions?

Next, ask your teen to do the same challenge.

Then, together, unpack and discuss what this means to you both, discover any gaps and encourage sharing observations, feelings, and concerns without judgment or expectations.

Hopefully, a level of clarity comes with this exercise and you gain more insight into the self-inquiry process, including your immediate needs, desires, and truths.

Reflections

I guarantee any unresolved or unhealed wounds from your own childhood or adolescence will be the source of your triggers while parenting a teen. There's just no getting around it. Just accept that your teen is born with the uncanny talent for zeroing in on those tender spaces inside of you and will continuously and unintentionally press into those wounds (with salty fingers no less), causing those old feelings to reactivate. We notice them through our reactions, our emotions, and old thought patterns rising to the surface. If our unhealed wounds and associated beliefs about ourselves remain unresolved, we are destined to pass these wounds down to our children. They will learn from your reactions and won't be able to help but internalize these experiences into their own stories of self. Raising emotionally healthy teens is dependent on your process of healing. Breaking generational wounds can begin with you.

One way for you to commit to your own healing is by cultivating a practice of reflection. Reflection is another form of self-inquiry and one of the most accessible ways to uncover and process your beliefs formed as a result of your childhood experiences.

Not all childhoods have big traumatic events, but even the most innocuous event in the mind of a child can be perceived as rejection, withdrawal, or not having their needs met. The repetition of those events can create "little traumas," which we'll talk about more in Chapter 5.

Reflecting on our own childhood experiences provides insights and reveals information we can piece together like a detective. When we are able to look at the original traumatic experiences from our childhood (both big and small) and reflect on the emotional scars, we can start distilling the disempowering beliefs that developed as a result of those experiences.

The human brain's natural response to any traumatic event is to make sense of it. This results in the creation of a flawed belief system about self, the world, and our relationship to it. If a traumatic experience happened in our childhood when we have a limited sense of the world, we may be unable to separate reality from perception, thus forming inaccurate beliefs about ourselves. For example, imagine the three-year-old version of you.

Imagine three-year-old you apologizing to one of your parents because you realize they had a really tough day at work and choose to honor that they don't have the mental capacity at that moment to sit on the floor and play Legos with you. No. That will never happen. The three-year-old you only knows what the three-year-old you wants and can only process based on their current developmental stage.

Reflecting on our own experiences as a child can help us recognize we did the best we could with the information we had at the time, appropriate to our developmental stage. Through reflections, we can start to see the beliefs we developed in response to these experiences (some traumatic, some not) are the root of our core beliefs, which limit and disempower us throughout our lifetime if they remain unchecked.

While I was writing this book, I reconnected with an old childhood friend. Growing up, we were the closest of friends and would spend countless hours together at each other's houses throughout our childhoods, adolescence, and early adulthood. She and I recalled many of the same memories and shared experiences. During this conversation, I asked her if she ever recalled witnessing any occasion when my mother was kind or affectionate towards me in any way. She couldn't remember a single occasion either.

I recognized my childhood experiences included feelings of abandonment, neglect, and lack of control. As a young child, I formed beliefs about who I was in order to make sense of these experiences. I internalized shame around believing I was unworthy, never good enough, and not worthy of love or kindness. I owned that belief because obviously, I was flawed, proving I was clearly not "enough." I couldn't argue with that when I had daily evidence to prove this belief, day in and day out.

As I entered my adolescence, my behavior changed, but my fundamental beliefs about myself did not. I developed a fierce sense of independence fueled by anger and rejection, which eventually turned into full-blown teen rebellion. My behavior was packed with acts of self-sabotage, drugs, sex, and, as I shared at the beginning of this chapter, running away from home. I started to use my voice and activate my own autonomy but not always in the healthiest ways.

All the experiences turned into trauma-informed beliefs about myself, which I carried with me throughout my life. I saw an abundance of evidence shown through my behavior, like my constant impulse to people-please or take care of others at my own expense, my need to be right, and so many more behaviors I'm not proud of. I recognized how deep my wounds ran, touching so many parts of myself.

As an adult, I desperately wanted to heal them for myself and for my son. Reflection helped, even though oftentimes it was extremely painful. Reflection, journaling, and self-healing are really big jobs.

Reflection through self-inquiry is the most common way to start this process, and journaling is a highly effective practice that helps to strengthen the communication between the conscious-thinking mind and the information stored deep within our subconscious mind. The act of reflection helps us understand how our emotional security developed and be able to look at those beliefs from the perspective of "now," not who we were as a child when those beliefs were formed. Some refer to this work as reparenting or shadow work.

One of the most powerful tools I found early in my self-directed healing journey was Byron Katie's "The Work." This is a tool I still use today in my own healing and with the teens I work with. I recommend you become familiar with her book *Loving What Is: Four Questions That Can Change Your Life,* as it is a wonderful way to start the process of self-inquiry. Byron Katie has made this tool freely available to download on her website, and she has published numerous YouTube videos of her facilitating "The Work" with other people. I have also included her book in the Suggested Reading section of this book and urge you to pursue this tool.

Briefly, Byron Katie's "The Work" consists of four questions and a "turnaround." The Work is simply as follows:

> Define the belief you are working with. Write it out or say it out loud with each step.
>
>> Question #1: Ask & Answer, "Is this true?"
>> Question #2: Ask & Answer, "Are you sure this is true?"
>> Question #3: Ask & Answer, "What do you feel when you think the thought _____?"
>> Question #4: Ask & Answer, "Who would you be without the thought _____?"

Then, the last part of the tool is to find five ways to turn the thought around. This is the reprogramming of the thought, allowing yourself to think, speak, and experience it from another perspective, causing a different firing sequence of the neurons. In this step, essential joy and playfulness are brought into the experience. Also, release the notion that the new way of experiencing the thought through the "turnaround" needs to contain truth.

The brain doesn't know what truth is, it just knows thoughts, which when habitually thought, have become beliefs.

Chapter 5: Fundamental Concepts

In the introduction, I shared my early passion for art. I even named my son after a painter I've always admired. I studied fine art in college and still dedicate a big portion of my time to painting and drawing. In college, the best piece of advice I received from a professor was to take the time to understand the fundamentals. Things like form, value, perspective, proportion, gesture, and more are the building blocks for most art.

Over the years I have studied many aspects of psychology, neurobiology, social issues, self-help, facilitation techniques, and learning and education topics in order to create a body of knowledge that ultimately helps me to support teens. This chapter is designed to take the most important fundamentals and distill them into palatable concepts to help you integrate this underlying knowledge into your own building blocks of understanding so you can better support your teen.

The Conscious, Preconscious & Unconscious Mind

Sigmund Freud is considered the grandfather of psychoanalytic theory. During his lifetime, his ideas were considered shocking and controversial by his contemporaries, yet his work had and continues to have a profound influence on a number of disciplines, including psychology, sociology, anthropology, literature, and even art.

While many of Freud's ideas have since fallen out of favor, one of his most important and enduring contributions to psychology is the theory of the conscious, preconscious, and unconscious mind. Many know this concept through his famous iceberg diagram. Freud believed behavior and thought were influenced by the unique interactions between those three domains, each operating on different levels of awareness.

Freud's Three Levels of Mind:

The Conscious Mind contains all of the thoughts, beliefs, memories, emotions, and desires we are aware of at any given moment. The conscious-thinking mind contains our awareness and rational thinking. This also includes our memories when we are thinking about them, which are not always part of consciousness but can be retrieved easily and brought into awareness.

The Preconscious Mind consists of anything that could potentially be brought into the conscious mind, like memories, thoughts, and beliefs.

The Unconscious Mind is the depository of feelings, thoughts, beliefs, urges, and memories that are outside of our conscious awareness. The unconscious contains contents that are unacceptable or unpleasant (often referred to as "shadows," which will be explored later in this chapter), such as feelings of pain, anxiety, or shame.

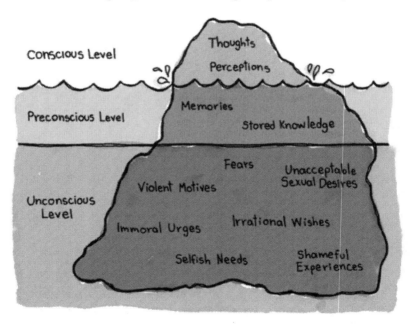

Freud analogized these three levels of the mind to an iceberg. The top of the iceberg poking out above the water represents the conscious mind. This is thought to be about 5% of the mind's processing awareness at any given time. The other 95% of activity resides under the surface of the water, often referred to as the subconscious and unconscious mind. Just below the conscious mind, we find the preconscious mind. However, the bulk of the iceberg is unseen beneath the waterline, which represents the depths of the unconscious mind.

Core Beliefs & Origins

Core beliefs are the many stories or narratives about ourselves derived from the past, our perceptions, our relationships, etc. Beliefs are practiced and grounded in our personal experiences. Many of these stories play in our minds like a favorite song set on repeat. Many times, these stories are playing without our knowledge and are ingrained into our subconscious minds. Whether the belief is true or fiction is unimportant to the brain, as the brain doesn't actually distinguish the difference between the two.

One job of the mind is to compute and make sense of the world. Simply put, this is done by taking our cumulative experiences, information learned, emotions, traumas (which we'll explore a little deeper in the next section), and outcomes and creating "stories." Sometimes the sense we make of the world doesn't make sense, but as a function of our mind, we have filled in the blanks, which is all happening within the subconscious mind.

The more we practice certain thought patterns, the more our brains become hardwired to default to firing the same neural pathways. This is how our habits are formed and behaviors are created. This is especially true if the thoughts activate our stress responses and create an internal turmoil, which can become a compulsive, emotional addiction. In other words, the more we think about something, the more we are likely to believe it, transforming thoughts into truths also called "core beliefs."

Core beliefs are not often questioned and play in the background as unnoticed music. Our thoughts become beliefs through interior and exterior validation, and they thrive. These core beliefs are, in essence, filters placed over the lens of how we view the world and ourselves, thus giving meaning to certain situations.

Whether we like it or not, some of our core beliefs about ourselves develop early in childhood. But in some respects, it feels like nature's cruel joke, since, in childhood, we are constrained by what we can cognitively understand based on biological developmental limitations. In childhood, we internalize our experiences and then translate them into messages in order to give meaning to our experiences. For example, when you were three years old, maybe your mother had a day when she was impatient with you. Maybe it was because she was busy, working from home, or on an important phone call. Through your three-year-old lens, you don't understand the separation between mom's other priorities and you.

To a toddler, all you feel is your needs not getting met at that moment, crucial attention is being withheld from you, and you feel the pain of dismissal. If your mother happened to use a sharp tone or raised her voice at you to wait, her words could have triggered your flight, fight, or freeze response, anchoring your experience with a strong emotional response. As a three-year-old, your brain may have internalized this situation as "I am bad," "I am not worthy of love," or "Something is wrong with me."

Why does the brain make these interpretations? During this stage of development, the toddler brain is processing the world through concepts of "me" and "mine." The toddler brain cannot grasp the concept of a separate life that mom is participating in outside of "me." The toddler brain can only function based on its current cognitive developmental stage, and the appropriate response to this situation, which may be anchored by strong emotion, is that there is something wrong with "me," therefore internalizing this experience into a story about self.

Guess what? We all have these core beliefs. Core beliefs are our foundational perceptions about our reality. Core beliefs inform the stories of "who I am," which run throughout our lives. Many of our core beliefs, unfortunately, are shaped by traumas both little and big from our childhood.

I have a vivid memory that shaped one of my core beliefs about myself, and it took me many years to heal and integrate. It doesn't mean this core belief is no longer there. It means that now, I can observe when it plays in my mind and choose an intentional response rather than reacting to it.

I was five years old, and my parents were hosting an adult dinner party with family, friends, and relatives. My bed was the designated place for people to put their handbags and coats. I was mingling around the living room with the guests and was so excited when I saw my grandmother walking down the hall from my bedroom. She was a beautiful woman, always so well put together, fashionable, and attractive. I remember giving her a big hug, and she whispered, "I've got a little something for you, and I'll give it to you later." Of course, my five-year-old self couldn't wait for later, so I headed back to my room to investigate.

There, on my bed, was a cotton jacket that perfectly matched the pattern of the lightweight sleeveless dress my grandmother was wearing. It was part of a set, very popular in the 1970s. In my five-year-old mind, it was my magical gift. It was a dress for me to wear so I could look like my beautiful grandmother. In my mind, it was the most magical gift a five-year-old girl who idolized her grandmother could receive. I put on her jacket, modeled it in the mirror, and concluded I looked as beautiful as my grandmother. I mustered up the confidence to go out into the living room where all the guests were mingling to show everyone how beautiful I was in that dress.

I entered the living room and announced, "Look what Granny brought me! I now look beautiful like her!"

At that moment, everyone's eyes were on me, and, almost as if a wave swept over the whole crowd, they all started laughing at once. They laughed and howled. I even caught my grandmother laughing at me.

My grandmother finally spoke up and said, "Lainie, that's my jacket, not a dress for you. Now, go and put that back in your room".

I returned to my room, removed her jacket, and felt so ashamed. I cried in my room and refused to come out and join the party for dinner saying that I had a "tummy ache." Throughout the evening, no one came in to check on me, except for my very annoyed mother who had to remove all of the coats and handbags on my bed and relocate them to her bed.

This incident developed and confirmed several core beliefs I had started to form about myself. At that moment, the brightness of my innocence and wide-eyed wonderment dimmed. I started to believe I was too much for people. I believed that if I was seen, I was going to be ridiculed and laughed at. In my mind, being too much for people also meant, in many respects, I wasn't good enough or worthy of being loved.

These are stories I've told myself all through adulthood. These are core beliefs that have influenced how I've interacted in personal relationships until I started to heal my core beliefs through shadow work (inner-child healing). When these core beliefs go unchecked in our lives, they affect everyone we interact with, including our children. As we parent our children, any unhealed traumas or wounds may be activated that lead us to recognize our deep-seated and unchallenged core beliefs. This is our work.

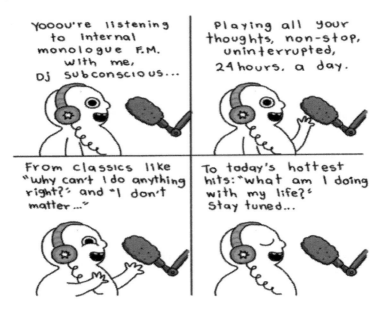

What are the stories you tell yourself?

Take a moment to check-in using self-inquiry and see if you can identify the stories you tell yourself.

Identify any of your own "I am _____" statements you've been telling yourself throughout your lifetime.

For the sake of this exercise, please look at the perceived negative ones. Are any of these familiar? "I am unlovable," "I am quick to anger," "I am too emotional," "I am not enough," "I am too much".
Once a belief is formed, our subconscious mind engages in what's called "confirmation bias" or, as I like to call it, filling in the gaps. In other words, information that does not confirm the belief is quietly ignored or discarded in preference for information that does.

In my case, since I had the core belief, "I am too much," I could subconsciously interpret my son's silence and non-response to my greetings, questions, or messages as "I am too demanding," therefore I'm really not valued or respected. When our core beliefs become activated, we see nothing but evidence to confirm this to be so, thus activating our inner wounds again and again and again.

Traumas

We've touched on traumas many times throughout this book already. Our unhealed traumas have a massive influence on who we are, how we see the world, and even how we parent. If you've never looked at these things before, this may be a little uncomfortable, but hey, this book is all about stepping outside of your comfort zone, right?

As a parent, it's our responsibility to identify, integrate, and heal these past traumas in order to support our teens. This section is designed to provide a fundamental understanding of what traumas are and how they affect our lives. If trauma is a large part of your or your teen's personal history, I suggest you pursue some of the resources listed in the Suggested Reading section.

What exactly are traumas? Traumas are patterns of thinking that are most commonly influenced by a specific event or series of events, which can be perceived as either big or small. The big traumas are the specific events you can identify, like getting dropped, having an accident, physical abuse, etc. Little traumas can have the exact same effect as the big traumas if they are repeated enough times, like the sound of an angry parent consistently slamming a door. Traumatic experiences stored as memories in the brain do not rely on time. The brain simply records that experience and unconsciously translates these experiences into beliefs about ourselves. Current and future sensory experiences that trigger the trauma wiring in your brain, as an example activated by a door slam, can also activate the meaning your subconscious assigned to that experience. Traumas are typically unresolved patterns in our subconscious minds, and our job is to unpack the stories we've created and integrate the thoughts to help us understand ourselves better.

There are two things you should consider about the subconscious mind in response to traumatic experiences.

First, the subconscious mind will try to create meaning out of the experience and try to make sense of it. If the subconscious mind needs to, it will fill in the blanks, create meaning where there may not have been, and lay the foundation for our core beliefs about ourselves, like we just explored. Traumas we've experienced in childhood tend to program our belief systems, something we will carry with us throughout our lives. The meaning our minds give to trauma is not necessarily based on logic, reasoning, or truth, rather it is based on making the best sense we can in the perception of our young minds.

Second, the subconscious mind will do whatever it can to try to keep you safe. Many times, staying safe looks like burying the original memory to prevent you from feeling pain. Some trauma responses will look like extreme behavior, like heightened focus on success, independence, achievement, etc. Other trauma responses may look like preventing yourself from doing self-inquiry work, meditation, journaling, or sharing your feelings with others. It's important to recognize the subconscious mind has one main objective – to keep you safe– and may view acts of self-inquiry as uncomfortable and potentially a threat.

I recently read a viral post shared on social media. This describes my personal trauma response experiences eloquently. Written by Jamila White of http://inspiredjamila.com/

> *This. Hits. Hard.*
>
> *The inability to receive support from others is a trauma response.*
>
> *Your "I don't need anyone, I'll just do it all myself" conditioning is a survival tactic. And you needed it to shield your heart from abuse, neglect, betrayal, and disappointment from those who could not or would not be there for you.*
>
> *From the parent who was absent and abandoned you by choice or the parent who was never home from working three jobs to feed and house you.*
>
> *From the lovers who offered sexual intimacy but never offered a safe haven that honored your heart.*
>
> *From the friendships and family who ALWAYS took more than they ever gave.*
>
> *From all the situations when someone told you "we're in this together" or "I got you" then abandoned you, leaving you to pick up the pieces when shit got real, leaving you to handle your part and their part, too.*
>
> *From all the lies and all the betrayals.*
>
> *You learned along the way that you just couldn't really trust people. Or that you could trust people, but only up to a certain point.*
>
> *Extreme-independence IS. A. TRUST. ISSUE.*
>
> *You learnt: if I don't put myself in a situation where I rely on someone, I won't have to be disappointed when they don't show up for me, or when they drop the ball... because they will ALWAYS drop the ball EVENTUALLY right?*
>
> *You may even have been intentionally taught this protection strategy by generations of hurt ancestors who came before you.*
>
> *Extreme-independence is a preemptive strike against heartbreak.*
>
> *So, you don't trust anyone.*

And you don't trust yourself, either, to choose people.
To trust is to hope, to trust is to be vulnerable.
"Never again," you vow.
But no matter how you dress it up and display it proudly to make it seem like this level of independence is what you always wanted to be, in truth it's your wounded, scarred, broken heart behind a protective brick wall.
Impenetrable. Nothing gets in. No hurt gets in. But no love gets in either.
Fortresses and armor are for those in battle, or who believe the battle is coming.
It's a trauma response.
The good news is trauma that is acknowledged is trauma that can be healed.
You are worthy of having support.
You are worthy of having true partnership.
You are worthy of love.
You are worthy of having your heart held.
You are worthy to be adored.
You are worthy to be cherished.
You are worthy to have someone say, "You rest. I got this."
And actually deliver on that promise.
You are worthy to receive.
You are worthy to receive.
You are worthy.
You don't have to earn it.
You don't have to prove it.
You don't have to bargain for it.
You don't have to beg for it.
You are worthy.
Worthy.
Simply because you exist.

- *Jamila White, @inspiredjamila*

As I've previously shared, my childhood was peppered with many traumas. I was raised by a parent who screamed at me frequently. As a child, my perception of this towering adult standing over me (even though she was a little woman in physical stature) screaming and yelling at me was a huge threat to my safety. Often, I would physically react by shaking with fear until I learned how to hide those responses. Even writing this now, here on this page, I feel tears welling up in my eyes, as this touches such a deep wound inside of me. Part of our challenge when we work on healing these past traumas is to acknowledge they may still carry an emotional charge. Imagine the unhealthy effects on you if you choose not to unpack these things and keep the emotion stored in your body instead. Guaranteed, that energy will discharge in some way.

I remember one instance of this happening to me vividly. It was a few years back in Peru, far removed from these childhood events. I was staying with a friend who was caring for his convalescent father. On one occasion, he was changing his father's catheter, and there turned out to be a giant mess, which I will spare you the details. He left that room, and in his anger, discharged those emotions by yelling and punching a wall. Even though it wasn't directed at me at all, I still jumped back and had visions of my mother standing over me and screaming. My body started shaking and I was transported into my youth in an instant.

We will never get rid of the history from these events, but we do need to acknowledge the history we are given and work with it so we can reprogram our auto-responses. This is why we do shadow work, or inner child work, as we will discuss in more detail later because our history will always be there. If we continue to let these triggers dictate our responses, then we are not helping our children. At the moment when one of these traumas is surfacing, instead of going into reaction mode and attacking the person who triggered you, be aware you are in that reactive state and use that awareness to choose an appropriate response.

From a biological perspective, trauma is an experience that causes the extreme activation of stress responses. This is true with any pattern of activating stress response systems that leads to an alteration of how that system functions, whether it be overactivity or reactivity. Prolonged activation of that pattern leads to the textbook definition of a trauma response.

Trauma should be examined through these 3 lenses:

- **Event:** The initial experience or circumstance— the thing that happened to cause the trauma. At the time, it could have been a single traumatic experience, but it could also be a cumulative response to many small experiences built up over time. Many times, the event may not be perceived as a big deal by an adult. Think of spilling milk on a carpet as a child. No matter how big or small it may have been, pinpointing the event can be important, but it is the least important of the three lenses.
- **Experience:** This is the compounded perception that we give to the event, either through the persistent consequences that came from it or the power we give it in our minds. Think of this as the accumulation of constantly getting yelled at in the milk spilling example above.
- **Effect:** How the event and experience affect the person in terms of their belief, the meaning they give to it. This meaning becomes a perception of how we view ourselves. In the same example, this would be like thinking you were a bad person for spilling milk on the rug.

Trauma prevents self-regulating, or the calm self, which is controlled by the prefrontal cortex. We'll go into the biology of the brain a little deeper in the next chapter. From a biological perspective, trauma causes the stress responses in our brains to fire. The fight, flight, or freeze responses are then triggered once our prefrontal cortex goes offline and the reptilian brain takes over. If you are unregulated, your stress responses are already activated. The more you recognize your triggers based on your traumas, the less challenging the present-day effects will be. You can use the trigger log in Chapter 4 to stay in tune with the things that are causing those traumas to resurface.

When people are faced with threats or prone to a lot of unpredictability, lack of control can activate the stress responses. Prolonged activation of those stress responses can then develop into trauma. Those who feel trauma do not feel safe and secure and thus cannot be creative or curious. In contrast, experiences with predictability, or moderate and controllable challenges, allow a person to develop deep resilience.

Commonly, trauma stems from a situation or environment where we have no control. We adapt by developing skills to create behaviors designed to help us get through childhood traumas. But as we get older, we are no longer as adaptive as we once were. This can be a telltale sign of patterned behaviors learned from childhood. This illustrates why it's so important to heal. Our work as parents is to look at our habitual behaviors in adulthood and heal the traumas, both big and little, through the lens of parenting. We are accountable.

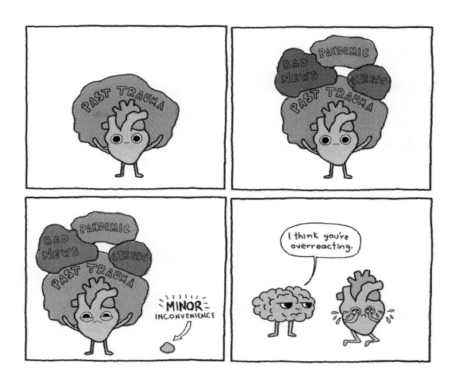

Love, belonging, joy, intimacy, and trust are all casualties of trauma. Those with unhealed traumas oftentimes do not have the ability to be vulnerable, which shuts down so many of those emotions. Trauma generates the habitual behavior of protection that creates layers of beliefs, emotions, and stories that need to be unpacked.

The COVID-19 pandemic is a collective trauma for parents and teens alike. This shared uncertainty and fear cause prolonged activation of stress responses. Now more than ever is the time to deal with our past traumas so we are more adept at pivoting to handle the new ones.

Shadows

"Everyone carries a shadow, and the less it is embodied in the individual's conscious life, the blacker and denser it is. At all counts, it forms an unconscious snag, thwarting our most well-meant intentions."
~ Carl Jung

There is a piece within each of us that we are afraid to show the world. Our hidden parts, which we deem unworthy, are cast into the shadows for fear of being exposed or others seeing this aspect of ourselves.

Carl Jung, a Swiss psychiatrist, is credited with influencing the way we think about the human psyche. Among many of his contributions to modern psychology, he is renowned for some of the best-known concepts, including synchronicity, archetypes (which we'll explore later in this chapter), introversion and extraversion, and "the shadow." Jung coined the term "shadow" to describe the hidden side of our psyche.

"The meeting with oneself is, at first, the meeting with one's own shadow. The shadow is a tight passage, a narrow door, whose painful constriction no

one is spared who goes down to the deep well. But one must learn to know oneself in order to know who one is."

~ Carl Jung

Exploring one's shadow and doing "shadow work" are popular practices within modern self-healing circles. There have been many books, workshops, and techniques developed over the last one hundred years, approaching healing through all sorts of different lenses, including but not limited to psychology itself. You will find some of my favorite resources in the Suggested Reading section of this book, and if you are on a self-healing path yourself, I highly recommend you pursue this particular fundamental.

Although the shadow is an innate part of the human experience, the vast majority are willfully blind regarding its existence. We cast our negative qualities in the darkness of our minds, hiding these qualities not only from others but from ourselves.

Our shadow beliefs are often revealed through psychological "projections," reflected in others. In other words, the things we see in other people that downright trigger us are revealing our own shadows. We often criticize and condemn others to ensure the focus does not fall on ourselves and reveal our own destructive tendencies. Many of us go through life with a false sense of moral superiority and believe we are wholly virtuous and generally in the right. It is our shadow that notices the actions of others and judges them as immoral, deficient, inferior, or wrong. To make things more complex, the shadow contains not just destructive aspects of the personality, but also positive, potent, creative, and powerful capabilities, which can be suppressed.

When our shadow remains unexplored in our unconscious mind, it can wreak havoc in our life. Repressed beliefs do not merely disappear, but rather they function independently outside of our conscious awareness. The shadow has the capacity to override our conscious-thinking mind and take possession of our perception, exerting control over our thoughts, feelings, and behavior. When our shadow takes over, we can be stuck in a pattern of thinking, looping over and over, causing self-destructive behaviors without our actual awareness.

So just where do our shadows come from?

Our shadows are created from our experiences and perceptions and are a part of the ongoing socialization process we participate in from birth. During our development, certain traits and impulses may have been condemned, not out of care but out of envy, fear, ignorance, or jealousy. These perceptions come from many places: our caregivers, early traumas, experiencing rejection of our impulses, and behaviors that misalign societal expectations. Our inclination to abide by certain social expectations can cause us to repress talents, innate abilities, and impulses that, if cultivated, have the potential to make us happier and more fulfilled. In Chapter 9, I share some tools to help your teen (and you) uncover the shadows through a series of exercises. But for now, set this book down, practice self-inquiry, and ask yourself, "What shadows have I been denying in my life?"

Shame

Shame and shadows are intrinsically linked. Often, shame is the glue that holds our shadows fixed deep within the depths of our subconscious minds. In this section, we will pull apart and examine the power shame has on our mental health. Shame is a powerful emotion that can potentially shape our lives in significant ways. Shame is defined as a condition of humiliating disgrace or disrepute.

Shame and guilt are commonly confused. The difference between shame and guilt is that guilt is a feeling experienced as a result of a behavior, while shame relates to how a person thinks about themselves. Oftentimes, these beliefs (habitually thought) become the person's identity, such as "I am unworthy," "I am disgraceful," "I am bad," etc.

Shame researcher Brené Brown Ph.D. says, "Shame is best defined as the intensely painful feeling or experience of believing we are flawed and therefore unworthy of acceptance and belonging." Brené Brown's works on this topic, including books, lectures, podcasts, and one of the most viewed talks in the world, the 2010 TED Talk "The Power of Vulnerability," are prolific.

"We judge people in areas where we're vulnerable to shame, especially picking folks who are doing worse than we're doing. If I feel good about my parenting, I have no interest in judging other people's choices. If I feel good about my body, I don't go around making fun of other people's weight or appearance. We're hard on each other because we're using each other as a launching pad out of our own perceived deficiency."
~ Brené Brown

People internalize shame for several reasons. Perhaps the most common precursor of shame is trauma. When something terrible happens to a person, they often feel a great deal of shame over what has happened. Sometimes these feelings are immediately internalized, tucked into the vaults of our subconscious.

Shame is built on foundations of fear, self-hatred, self-loathing, and oftentimes, the belief that you are not "enough." Shame works with the shadows to hide and reject the parts of ourselves we believe others will judge and deem unworthy. When a person feels ashamed of themselves, they may struggle to find a sense of worthiness, and oftentimes shame is linked to a person's self-esteem.

Shame can impact the whole trajectory of a person's life.

Here are five ways shame shapes peoples' lives. See if you can recognize any of these traits within yourself or your teen:

1. Often people with shame will avoid vulnerability and rarely share their true selves with the world. This may look like isolating themselves and avoiding relationships, vulnerability, and community.

2. Often people with shame tend to keep their thoughts and emotions to themselves and practice suppressing their feelings.

3. Often people who feel ongoing shame are commonly living out difficult emotional and mental challenges, which can lead to depression, anxiety, and the effects of low self-esteem.

4. Often, adolescents (and adults) who have an omnipresent sense of shame are less likely to take healthy risks or step outside of their comfort zones for fear of being judged by others. The fear of being devalued, judged, or failing outweighs the healthy risks one must take in order to grow.

5. Often, people who live with shame are more likely to gravitate towards self-destructive behaviors. Feelings of shame and unworthiness can result in not choosing a path of healing.

"If we are going to find our way out of shame and back to each other, vulnerability is the path and courage is the light. To set down those lists of *what we're supposed to be* is brave. To love ourselves and support each other in the process of becoming real is perhaps the greatest single act of daring greatly."

~ Brené Brown

In her book, *The Gifts of Imperfection*, Brené Brown writes about the keys to overcoming shame by developing something she calls "shame resilience." Shame resilience means being able to identify shame as it occurs and move past it in healthy ways. For example, shame resilience may involve challenging the self-critical thoughts that shame triggers or evaluating the validity of your shame. This is really an act of being the watcher of your thoughts and immediately applying self-inquiry.

According to Brown, here are the steps to develop shame resilience:

1. Recognize how shame manifests in you, where you physically feel it in your body, what emotions pop up, and which thought patterns (beliefs) are linked.
2. Spend some time identifying and evaluating the root causes of your shame through self-inquiry. Name the causes, expectations, and judgments you are practicing in your mind as this feeling of shame is activated.
3. Challenge social and societal messages that equate flaws with inadequacy or unworthiness. Recognize when you are holding yourself to the standards of perfection and allow yourself to accept your mistakes.
4. Open up and confide in someone trustworthy about your shame. Both shadows and shame rely on secrecy in order to have power over your life. Talking about shame removes its hold on you and helps you step into vulnerability and connection.

The way to overcome the hold shame has on us is to build trusted relationships through vulnerability. Keep this in mind when you work on healing your own shame and set out to support your teen with theirs.

Archetypes

Archetypes are a tool to help us answer the question, "Who am I?"

This is a question all adolescents struggle with. In fact, it's a question most adults continue to address throughout their lives, but the questioning and exploring begin early in adolescence. Answers to this question go deeper than the obvious (I am a daughter, a sister, etc.). During adolescence, young people are wired to try on different identities, sometimes one after another, as part of a natural process of discovery. Identity exploration is hardwired into humans. Keep in mind, during the teen years, identity exploration is influenced by many factors, including social status, which has a great impact on their exploration.

One of the ways humans explore identities is through what Carl Jung calls "archetypes." According to Jung, archetypes are defined as common pattern structures or symbols inherent to the human psyche. In fact, Jung postulates that archetypes are the psychic counterpart of instinct, described as unconscious cultural knowledge, responsible for guiding conscious behavior.

Some might refer to archetypes as pseudoscience, but like many of the other concepts we have spoken about in this book, this is yet another tool or framework to help you explore, understand, and support your adolescents. Take it or leave it, but from personal experience, facilitating archetype work with teens is a very effective way to encourage deeper self-inquiry and exploration.

Archetypes can be found and traced throughout most cultures and time periods present in historical writings, myths, fables, legends, fairy tales, origin stories, and oral history. Jung identifies twelve main archetypes, but variations can be found in other systems as well – all with merit. The twelve we'll outline here are:

1. **The Sage:** A free thinker. Their intellect and knowledge are their reason for living, their essence. They seek to understand the world and their being by using their intelligence and analytical skills. They always have a fact, a quote, or a logical argument on the tip of their tongue.

2. **The Innocent:** They seem to have read and absorbed every self-help book in the world. They're optimistic and always searching for happiness. The innocent sees the good in everything. They want to feel well-adjusted to the world around them. The innocent also wants to please others and feel like they belong.

3. **The Explorer:** A bold traveler. They set out without a clear path and are always open to novelty and adventure. The explorer has a deep love of discovering new places and new things about themselves. The

downside of the explorer archetype is that they're always searching for perfection, and they're never satisfied.

4. **The Ruler:** A classic leader. They believe they should be the ones to bring order to any situation. The ruler is stable, strives for excellence, and wants everyone to follow their lead. They tend to have plenty of reasons why everyone should listen to them. This is one of the 12 Jungian archetypes related to power. The ruler, in their desire to impose their will on others, can easily become a tyrant.

5. **The Creator:** Has a profound desire for freedom because they love novelty. They love to transform things in order to make something completely new. The creator is clever, non-conformist, and self-sufficient. They're imaginative and good-humored. However, they can also be inconsistent and spend more time thinking than actually doing.

6. **The Caregiver:** Feels stronger than other people. Consequently, they offer maternal protection to those around them. They want to protect people from harm and try to prevent any danger or risk from threatening other people's happiness. In extreme cases, the caregiver turns into a martyr who constantly reminds everyone of their sacrifices.

7. **The Magician:** Like a great revolutionary. They regenerate and renew not just for themselves, but for others as well. They're constantly growing and transforming. The negative side of the magician archetype is that their mood can be contagious. They sometimes turn positive events into negative ones.

8. **The Hero:** The axis of a hero's life is power. The hero has an uncommon vitality and resistance that they use to fight for power or honor. They'll do anything to avoid losing. In fact, they don't lose because they never give up. The hero can be overly ambitious and controlling.

9. **The Rebel:** A transgressor. They provoke people and don't care at all about other people's opinions. As a result, they like going against the grain and thinking for themselves. They don't like to be pressured or influenced. The negative side to the rebel archetype is that they can become self-destructive.

10. **The Lover:** All heart and sensitivity. They love, love, and love to lavish it on other people. Their greatest happiness is feeling loved. They enjoy everything that's pleasing to the senses. They value beauty (in every sense of the word) above all.

11. **The Jester:** Likes to laugh, even at themselves. They don't wear any masks and tend to break down other people's walls. They never take themselves seriously because their goal is to enjoy life. The negative side of the jester is that they can be lewd, lazy, and greedy.

12. **The Orphan:** They walk around with open wounds. They feel betrayed and disappointed. They want other people to take charge of their life. When no one does, they feel disappointed. They tend to spend time with people who feel just like them. The orphan often plays the victim. They pretend to be innocent. The orphan has a cynical side and manipulative talent.

Think about archetypes as a framework containing symbolic personalities. This framework is expressed slightly differently throughout time based on the culture or time period. But if you look deep enough, you'll notice there are always common threads. For example, the ruler archetype in modern-day America may be personified through your lens as Obama or Trump, depending on your own political views. You can also identify some similar qualities in Zeus by looking at the ruler archetype from Ancient Greek mythology. Clearly, there are lots of differences as well, but the common thread, archetypal personality, is what we are identifying with, and this provides all cultures of all ages an inherent understanding of the world around us.

Within Jung's theory, archetypes reside in an area of the psyche called the collective unconscious. The belief is that all humans are born with a general ancestral memory or knowledge of these archetypes, and we each have access to them when they are needed.

The role archetypes play in our own personal evolution is to provide each one of us access to tools to support our development. Furthermore, children commonly access this information through exploration and play, allowing them to step into roles and embody the archetype itself. When a child is playing make-believe and pretending to be a pirate, a princess, or a doctor, essentially what they are doing is experimenting with identities and social masks and exploring aspects of these archetypes.

I'm sure you've witnessed your own children construct limitless games around anything and everything led by their imagination. I've watched my son with a group of his friends transform into lions, and each child stepped into self-assigned roles. I've witnessed the king lion sit on his throne and rule the jungle. I've observed a little girl seamlessly step into the role of the mom lioness and care for her cubs. Another little boy became an explorer and led an expedition deep into the imaginary dense jungle, setting out for an adventure. The role-playing game went on for hours as I watched them morph into new characters, sets of circumstances, and ultimately new roles and challenges to overcome. This is an example of instinctual play, a child's way of feeling out and exploring many personalities and archetypes.

As children grow into teenagers, they start to construct more complex identities. As a parent, you may notice more of these archetypes explored through imitation and identification with various role models. If your teen has role models, follows certain influencers, or gravitates towards certain styles of music, they may be identifying with the archetype of that person or the personality of the music. For example, does this musical genre follow the framework of the Jester, the Magician, or the Hero? Perhaps it is a combination of them all or something else entirely.

Using the archetypes as a tool to explore these ideas helps you learn more about your teen and helps your teen understand themselves a little better. A great way to encourage your teen to begin thinking about archetypes is by challenging them to identify which archetype their favorite celebrities most resemble.

An important aspect to understanding archetypes is recognizing that each person has access to all these archetypes as a tool. They can be seen as masks to help each one of us borrow the strength, will, or identity of our shared human psyche to help us work through certain challenges. Time to take closer notice and recognize if your teen is strongly identified with one of these archetypes. Is this identification causing them to suppress other aspects within themself? By nature, masking has both positive and negative effects, and when exploring concepts of archetypes, the key point is balance and recognizing there is a nuanced difference between putting on a mask and hiding behind one.

Attachment Theory

Attachment theory was developed by British psychiatrist John Bowlby in the 1960s. The theory explores how our brains are wired to help us thrive and survive in the environment we were born into. Over the past 50 years, researchers have explored how to predict and explain children's behavior by understanding their attachment styles.

Learning about attachment theory and attachment styles is an important fundamental to understanding ourselves better and creating a more connected relationship with our teens. Attachment styles influence so much of who we are, what our default patterns are, and how we relate to the world.

In order to support our teens, we need to take a closer look at the quality of our relationships. If we find ourselves stuck repeating patterns in our relationships (with our teens, other family members, colleagues, and friends), we can feel helpless, overwhelmed, frustrated, and disparaged. A good way to understand the dynamics that play out in our relationships is to look closer at our behaviors through the lens of our attachment style.

There are three primary characteristics that help determine which attachment style you are dominantly operating with. Most people identify with a particular attachment style, but that does not mean you will never display qualities or attributes of other styles. Please use honest reflection and self-inquiry as you think about how the following characteristics show up in your life. Use a journal or the Notes section at the end of this book to write your reflections as you consider how the following three characteristics have shown up in your life.

1. Consider comfort and intimacy as a characteristic. How comfortable are you? How comfortable have you been throughout your life being in close relationships, intimate, and vulnerable with others?

2. Think about your relationship between dependence and avoidance. To what extent do you feel comfortable depending on others and having people depend on you?

3. Do you often experience anxiety that shows up as worry that your partners, significant others, family close friends, or peers will abandon and reject you?

Addressing our attachment styles requires self-inquiry, self-awareness, and a willingness to contextualize our emotional responses and memories objectively. The key is to notice patterns that come up in our lives, even if long ago we wrote those situations off as a coincidence. Examine the lingering strong emotions that remain in those memories and try to recognize if there are any signs that you've inadvertently sabotaged your relationships in any way.

One of the great things about reflection is that it gives us the opportunity to notice our own behaviors as a contributor to lifelong patterns. If we notice the same patterns have repeated in our relationships and we have had trouble getting our needs met, this is an indicator that there may be a need to go deeper inward and heal.

Attachment patterns can be passed down from one generation to the next. Children learn how to connect from their parents and caregivers, and they in turn model this way of connecting to the next generation. Your attachment history, which creates your attachment style, plays a crucial role in how you relate to your children. Understanding your own attachment patterns will help you to develop awareness and accountability and notice your beliefs based on your own early childhood wiring.

The four attachment styles are:

- **The Secure Model:** This is a relationship wherein the child has had a consistent sense of being seen, heard, soothed, and an overall feeling of safety from the parent/parents. This style is low on avoidance and anxiety. Those with this style are comfortable with intimacy; not worried about rejection or preoccupied with the relationship. It is easy for them to get close to others and feel comfortable depending on them and vice versa. They don't worry about being abandoned or about someone getting too close.

- **The Avoidant Model:** This is a relationship wherein the child has been neglected, unheard, or unseen by one or both parents and can result in resentment toward both or one of the parents. This style is high on avoidance and low on anxiety. Those with this style are uncomfortable with closeness and primarily value independence and freedom; not worried about their partner's availability. They find it difficult to trust and depend on others and prefer others do not depend on them. It is very important for them to feel independent and self-sufficient.

- **The Ambivalent Model:** This is a relationship of uncertainty and unreliability where the child never consistently feels safe, seen, or heard. This attachment style typically comes from the separation of parents. This style is low on avoidance and high on anxiety. Those with this style crave closeness and intimacy and are very insecure about the relationship. They want to be extremely emotionally close, even merge, with others, but others are reluctant to get as close as they might like. They often worry their partner doesn't love or value them and will abandon them. Their inordinate need for closeness scares people away.

- **The Disorganized Model:** This is when the parents or primary caregivers have provided terrifying experiences for a child, either from a child taking on the parents' fear or by being physically or verbally abusive. This leads to a disassociated child, who cannot handle their emotions and constantly acts out or pushes people away. This style can occur in the context of the other three insecure models. There are two things going on in the brain when this model is in play. One is the ancient brainstem circuit that mediates a survival reaction, namely fight, flight, or freeze. The second circuit is a limbic-based attachment system that provides motivation. Those with this model are torn between going towards and away from the cause of their disorganization at the same time.

The descriptions above are a basic guideline to help you understand the dominant patterns in your life. However, many people can demonstrate attributes of more than one attachment model. Just as each of us is unique, so is our attachment model programming. If you are having a difficult time determining your attachment style based on the information above, there are numerous online tests and quizzes to help you. Just do a search. Also, there are countless books available on attachment theory, and I've included a robust section for your reference in the Suggested Reading section of this book.

Once you understand your own attachment style, you will be able to predict your likely response in different circumstances. For example, if you have an avoidant attachment style, your fear of rejection may override your desire to be promoted at work, and you may pull yourself out of the running for consideration. By recognizing your fear of rejection as an old habit based on your early childhood programming, you can overcome the obstacles by consciously taking steps to shift your mindset. Taking positive steps can help you rewire your brain and develop a more secure attachment style.

As someone who is committed to parenting in partnership with your teen, it's vital to recognize that your self-esteem, your ability to control your emotions, and the quality of your relationships are all affected by your attachment style. Remember, you are accountable for the "you" you bring to the relationship. Recognize from the exercise above that your attachment style will influence the following:

- How you perceive and deal with closeness and emotional intimacy.
- Your ability to communicate your emotions and needs and listen to and understand the emotions and needs of your teens.
- How you respond to conflict and uncomfortable conversations.
- What expectations you have of your teens. (Remember, expectations are relationship killers.)

After reading the descriptions of the attachment styles and knowing what you know about my story, you might have guessed, my brain developed a disorganized attachment model, but throughout my life, I've demonstrated attributes of both the ambivalent and avoidant models as well.

My attachment style informed many of the problems in my adult relationships until I started to recognize what was going on. I noticed a pattern of pulling those around me close, then when I felt threatened, I would push them away for no reason. That was a familiar pattern I learned from my childhood, and I couldn't help it. My brain was wired to act out this way. Bring them close, push them away, bring them close, push them away. This behavior always produced the same result: they finally retreated. This reinforced some of my core beliefs, like "Everyone leaves," "I'm not worthy of being loved," or "No one sees, hears, or understands me."

If we don't resolve these destructive patterns in ourselves, they will flow into all our relationships, including those with our teens. As we've discussed before, adolescents have the uncanny talent for knowing exactly how to trigger you, and your reaction can be predicted if you haven't taken the time to unpack these patterns and heal yourself. This is one of the reasons identifying the patterns in your relationships will help you to recognize how your brain is programmed and move towards healing.

As you start to explore your own attachment wounds, you must commit to removing blame. Remember, none of us have control over the ways we were raised. The best we can do as adults is make an effort to understand our own stories and use that information to grow as people (and parents). Exploring attachment theory can be tough, especially if it means unpacking painful memories from your childhood or past relationships. But awareness of our attachment style can make us more self-aware.

When we know our triggers from our attachment wounds, we can find ways to work through our emotions, communicate better, and navigate or set boundaries more effectively. If you are committed to healing and becoming securely attached, the way you treat your children will shift through that awareness.

Childism

Talking about childism can be challenging, triggering, and an uncomfortable reality check for any parent. I have included this topic in my book not to shame any parent who has never broached the topic before now, but to empower you with information to help you question your own beliefs.

Elizabeth Young-Bruehl defines childism in her book *Childism: Confronting Prejudice Against Children* as, "a prejudice against children on the grounds of a belief that they are property and can (or even should) be controlled, enslaved, or removed to serve adult needs."

Most adults who have never considered childism have likely never looked at their own inherent prejudices against children and the blind acceptance that children should have a limited role in a society dominated by adults. Childism is the hardest form of prejudice to recognize because children are the one group that is naturally subordinate until they reach the age of "consent." In our culture, parents are the responsible party and have custody of their children, which can also be looked at as ownership, negating the rights of the child based on the desires, rules, and control of the adult.

Most people don't consciously or actively practice childism through the lens of ownership, but there can be subtle beliefs inherent in our parenting practices that lean towards authoritarianism. Many of these habits are ingrained inside of us as parents. By the time our children reach adolescence, we have already been practicing some form of childism for a very long time.

See if you can recognize some of the consequences or signs of childism in your own life.

- Children or adolescents are expected to conform to adults' timetables and expectations.

- Children or adolescents are conditioned to think authority has the right to judge them. (Am I good, right, appropriate, etc.?)

- It's common practice or acceptable to patronize or talk down to children or adolescents.

- Adults talk over the heads of children or adolescents.

- Adults laugh at our children or adolescents' failures, mistakes, or misdeeds on social media.

- Adults hold their children and adolescents to higher standards of self-regulation than they do themselves. (We are allowed to "vent," but when kids throw fits, temper tantrums, or give us the silent treatment, we find this unacceptable and disrespectful.)

- Adults object to any show of their child or adolescent's autonomy. (Adults can have dietary preferences, but a child is called a picky eater.)

- Adults impose behavior modification techniques, such as punishments and rewards, on their children or adolescents.

- Adults value quiet obedience and conformity above individuality and freedom.

- Children become targets of adults based on adults' unresolved trauma.

The point of this section is to help you pull apart some of those unquestioned beliefs that may come in between you and your adolescence with the goal of eliminating the blocks preventing you from connecting respectfully and authentically with your teen.

Social Learning Theory

Isolation is the nemesis of the teen brain. The brain is wired to start individuating from the family unit at around this point in the developmental process. One of the ways it does this is by creating a greater sense of learning from the peer group and figuring out how they fit into the world. The thought of pulling away from family identity is what they are wrestling with.

Social groups are important for humans of all ages as evidenced by Maslow's hierarchy of needs, but they are a much bigger part of the teen experience. It is also important to note that Maslow's framework, much like psychology and neuroscience as a whole, has been modified multiple times over the years. As with any principle in this book or in life in general, if something doesn't work for you, toss it out. The understanding and individual lessons we can learn from the concepts are far more important than buying into the work as a whole.

With that said, Maslow believed those in isolation are frustrated and don't understand why. It occurs because they are longing for social connection as they transform from being dependent on others to an individual of their own design. Social learning creates a desire to fit in. Teens are now starting to think about what group they want to be associated with and the feelings that come with the fear of not fitting in with them. For young children, friends and social circles are often determined by factors outside of their control, such as who lives close by or who parents choose to let inside their own social circles.

It can be overwhelming for teens to try and figure out where they fit on the social spectrum as they become more aware of other people their age they may not have been exposed to before. This is the age where teens are able to reflect on their own identity through those in their peer group. The social aspect is as important for their own inward growth as it is for outward development.

There are many benefits to having control over one's own social structure, especially in these developmental years. Hearing about the struggles of other teens can normalize self-development and help peers understand they are not alone in the process. The brain is very receptive to this growth at this time, and it is seeking out new sources to learn from. This doesn't mean the family unit is any less important. Instead, it means there is merely not enough variety of stimulation there to help broaden teens' horizons.

Another benefit to social learning is in finding outlets for expression by fulfilling roles and trying new identities they cannot at home. Maybe your teen wants to be a leader and take charge of certain situations, but they have older siblings who do not allow this experience. In a new social group, teens can be whatever they want to be. The young person is literally creating the persona of who and what they want to be amongst peers who have no reason to see them as anything different.

Dr. Daniel Siegel goes into much greater detail to explain exactly why all of this happens. In one of his speeches, Siegel reminds us that adolescence is not just about impulsivity and risk-taking. There are physical changes in the brain causing hyper-rational thinking and changes in dopamine. Although adolescents may be separating from their parents, they move towards forming deeper relationships with their peers. Just like other mammals, humans find safety in groups and surrounding ourselves with peers allows us to survive. When we see adolescents desperately seeking to fit in, this is part of the brain's natural instincts, not just over-dramatic teen behavior. When teens don't feel like they are part of a group, they experience a sense of urgency and of life and death.

I'm sure you've heard your teen say something like, "I need to have this brand of shoe, all my friends have them" or "I need to have a new outfit," or "I have to go to that party". You don't necessarily need to buy the shoe or the outfit or let them go to the party, but as parents, we can at least understand the feeling of their suffering in an empathic way. We can understand their point of view and how this life-or-death feeling is not something they're just making up because they're caving into peer pressure. It can be from millions of years of evolution basically built into your DNA, telling you if you're an adolescent, you should be a member of at least a friendship, if not a larger group.

Now, the downside of this social engagement process is you can forsake morality for the benefit of membership, and that's called peer pressure. The positive side of this social engagement is you learn social skills that can last a lifetime. The friendships you develop can teach you how to be connected to other people when the self is not living in isolation. All the studies of well-being, from mental and medical well-being to longevity happiness, show relationships are a primary factor allowing you to achieve all those positive states within. We have seen how the dopamine changes drive you to experience new things and how hyper-rational thinking also pushes in that direction. And so, we can see that novelty is built into what the adolescent experience is all about.

Learning from each other is human nature, and it begins from the moment we are born. As social creatures, we discover new things all the time through observation, demonstration, imitation, and the sharing of knowledge and direct experience. When we come together as a group, the learning potential is exponential. According to Albert Bandura's social learning theory, learning is a cognitive process that takes place in a social context and can occur purely through observation or direct instruction.

From a behavioral standpoint, the evolution of social learning theory attempts to explain human behavior in terms of continuous reciprocal interaction between cognitive, behavioral, and environmental influences. In other words, we learn from each other through observation and modeling — experiencing someone's behavior, ideas, skills, or perspective and adopting them as our own. This helps to explain how babies and young children model the actions and behaviors, both negative and positive, of the adults in their lives. It also accounts for cultural intelligence and influence, as well as fads and trends, from everything to fashion to technology to popular music.

Social learning theory is a generalized psychological explanation of behavioral learning. It can be applied to any situation where people have the opportunity to influence each other. When we share our experiences within a group, two things occur. We allow for the process of osmosis, where others in the group have the opportunity to learn from us, to literally absorb information and ideas. We also have the opportunity to foster empathy in others by sharing our feelings and our perspective on important life issues.

143

Chapter 6: Adolescent Brain Biology Basics

Do you sometimes act before thinking? What about your teen? Are they often impulsive? Have you ever wondered why? Do you worry about the consequences of their actions even if they don't seem to? If you answered "yes" to any of these questions, this chapter will help you understand why.

Imagine your finger is ready to hit "send" as your eyes scan the angry text comeback you've drafted to your teen. Some of the things you've written are really harsh and maybe a little unfair. In a flash, you reconsider and revise your text to calm your tone.

Now, imagine the situation is reversed. You said or did something to piss off your teen. They respond quickly without hesitation. Their words sting. Somewhere tucked deep inside of them they may have realized they probably shouldn't have hit send, but their brain flashes with anger or annoyance, and they just couldn't help themselves. Their message cuts into you deep, and you wish you didn't read what they just wrote.

Impulsive decisions – acting before thinking about the consequences – happen more often in teens than in adults. But let's be clear, adults aren't immune to rash decisions either. In this chapter, we'll unpack the biological and physiological reasons behind what's going on.

Biology and psychology have been around for ages, but the concepts are constantly being refined. Throughout this chapter, we are going to reference several experts. Their research and findings may not be totally accepted by every scientist, researcher, and doctor on the planet, but the underlying principles draw from widely accepted norms. Understanding neurobiology in the adolescent brain is important because it frames how the parent views their activity. They are not doing whatever they do to intentionally annoy you, at least not most of the time (I hope). In many cases, their actions are a byproduct of the biological and psychological changes taking place in their brains.

The Biology of Decision-Making

First, we are going to explore the biology of decision-making in the brain. Making decisions isn't necessarily an act of the conscious mind nor does it happen without biological processes. Decisions require a series of events to happen within the brain, all of which happen within a fraction of a second.

Decision-making relies on different neural clusters communicating with each other by way of electrochemical impulses and chemical messengers, called neurotransmitters. These structures are made up of specialized cells called neurons.

Decision-making requires teamwork among these specialized structures in the brain to analyze the information flowing through them in order to process a response. As I said, this process is instantaneous and relies on each brain structure and system to do its part. The response or output provides the basis for our behaviors and actions.

The process of decision-making in an adult brain and within a teen's brain is basically the same, but there are slight differences. We know the adolescent brain is not fully developed until its early twenties. This means the way the adolescents' decision-making circuit integrates and processes information may put them at a disadvantage. Although the brain may have grown to its full adult size by early teens, regions of the brain continue to mature until the age of about twenty-five. One of the brain regions that matures later is the prefrontal cortex. Basically, the prefrontal cortex is the control center, tasked with thinking ahead and evaluating consequences, risks versus rewards. The prefrontal cortex is the area of the brain responsible for preventing you from sending off that initial angry text to your teen and modifying it with kinder words.

While the brain's prefrontal cortex matures later, the limbic system matures earlier. The limbic system plays a central role in processing emotional responses. Because of its earlier development, the limbic system is more likely to influence decision-making. What does this mean? Decision-making in the adolescent brain is led by emotional charges more than the perception of consequences. Naturally, there is an imbalance between feeling-based decision-making ruled by the more mature limbic system and logical-based decision-making by the not-yet-mature prefrontal cortex. This may explain why teens are more likely to make "bad" decisions, such as drugs, alcohol, and other risky behavior, (more of which we'll explore in the next chapter).

Let's look at this a little closer. Over the years, researchers have thoroughly explored the consequences of this imbalance in the adolescent brain as compared to the fully developed adult brain. In one fascinating study, adolescents and adults were shown the same set of photographs of faces of people, of all ages, races, ethnicities, genders, etc., while recording the brain activity of both groups. However, each of the photographs used in this study were of people who had what were considered "neutral expressions." The same photographs were shown to the adults and the adolescents while recording which part of their brains activated when looking at the photos. The same photo that activated the adult's reasoning prefrontal cortex caused the emotional amygdala of the teen brain to light up like a Christmas tree. The conclusion was that the adolescent perceives the neutral expression through the lens of emotions driven by the limbic system and sees hostility, aggression, or any other number of emotions.

Think about the implications. Your teen's lower limbic system is working full-time. What happens when you innocently make a remark about a project your teen is working on? (Cue teen's emotional reaction.) What happens when you ask how their day was? ("Why are you grilling me?") What reaction do you get when you ask for help with the dishes? (A sigh.) How do they respond when you ask how a certain friend is? (Eye roll.) How many times have you thought your teen was overreacting? How many times have you been on the receiving end of their anger or "attitude," the slammed door, or their dismissal? Knowing what you now know about the lower limbic system, recognize theirs is working perfectly fine, and please don't take their reactions personally. They are wired to be offended, emotional, and "rude." Whether you like it or not, you are the perfect person to be on the receiving end.

Remodeling of the Teen Brain

Like the rest of the body, the brain will reach peak performance as it matures. Throughout adolescence, the brain is busy fine-tuning itself through two key processes: myelination and synaptic pruning, which we briefly touched upon in Chapter 3.

Neurons are surrounded by branch-like structures called dendrites and thread-like fibers called axons. Dendrites bring information into the neurons, while axons transport info out of the neuron and pass the information along the circuitry. Each dendrite will see the connection of a surrounding neuron's axon to create a puzzle-like connection throughout the system. The small space between the axon and the neuron, where a signal travels and information is exchanged, is called a synapse.

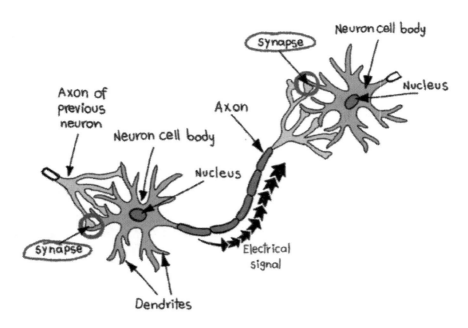

As the adolescent brain matures, this neutral circuitry starts to optimize through a process called myelination, which supports the brain to process information faster and more reliably. In myelination, axons wrap themselves in a fatty substance called a myelin sheath, which works like plastic insulation around electrical wires. This boosts the brain's efficiency by increasing the speed at which a signal travels down the axon by up to 100 times. Think of this as a "superhighway" with a long stretch of road without any off-ramps. This superhighway has been optimized for speed and efficiency.

Myelinated circuits are 3,000 times more coordinated and quicker. These "superhighways" allow the whole system to work in a much more effective way. As new highways are being paved through myelination, they block access to off-ramps not used that often. In this metaphor, the off-ramps refer to synapses or previous connections between one neuron and another. The blocking off these connections is called "pruning." With synaptic pruning, synapses are removed, allowing the brain to redirect precious resources toward more active synapses.

The adolescent brain is literally reconstructing itself and the way it thinks. New deeper connections are made as the brain is reshaping and remodeling itself in response to your teen's focus, experiences, and activities.

I bet you are wondering, "how does the dominant limbic system affect your teen's adolescent experience?" I bet you can characterize the way you perceive your teen through these two words: ***emotional intensity.***

Sometimes you notice your teen, perhaps in the company of other teens, filled with laughter, hysterics, and heightened joy. Other times, you characterize your teen caught in a cycle of lows and your very presence, as a source of their annoyance, causing angst, sarcasm, rudeness, or a full-blown shutdown. Whichever end of the spectrum they are embodying, the emotional intensity is the consistent thread.

Another byproduct of the dominant limbic system is that adolescents tend to gravitate toward the unfamiliar. Just as we explored, teens can easily make choices that may be unsafe. Traditionally, risk-taking behaviors in teens have been analyzed from a psychopathological approach. However, from an evolutionary theory, many researchers believe risk-taking is actually a means through which adolescents obtain potential benefits for survival and reproduction. In simpler words, risk-taking prepares the young person for adulthood.

While we are considering adolescent behavior, let's reframe our understanding into a positive appreciation. The ease with which teens can access emotional intensity is a gift. This quality helps humans access enthusiasm for life, our ability to be present, and an unabridged capacity to feel our way through the world. Think about it this way, adolescence is a great time to take risks, especially if they feel safe, grounded, and in partnership with their parents. Remembering this emotional intensity can serve us to rekindle our own zest for life since many of us have dulled or repressed this natural ability within ourselves as adults.

In his book *Brainstorm The Power and the Purpose of the Teenage Brain*, Dr. Daniel Siegel explores the psychological aspects of emotional intensity in teens. He uses the acronym "ESSENCE" to explain the four key qualities happening within the adolescent brain.

According to Siegel, there are four vital features to adolescence that we can all, whatever age we may be, cultivate, these are:

ES: Emotional Spark – honoring these important internal sensations, which are more intense during adolescence, serve to create meaning and vitality throughout our lives.

SE: Social Engagement – the important connections we have with others that support our journeys through life with meaningful, mutually rewarding relationships.

N: Novelty (Doing something new) – how we seek out and create new experiences that engage us fully, stimulating our senses, emotions, thinking, and bodies in new and challenging ways.

CE: Creative Exploration – the conceptual thinking, abstract reasoning, and expanded consciousness that create a gateway to seeing the world through new lenses.

The Hand Brain Model

Dr. Dan Siegel developed the "hand brain model." This model is a powerful tool that has helped children, adolescents, and their caregivers conceptualize what happens in the brain, specifically during times of dysregulation. Having the language to articulate our biological reactions is helpful for so many reasons, including enhancing the ability to regulate our own emotions through awareness.

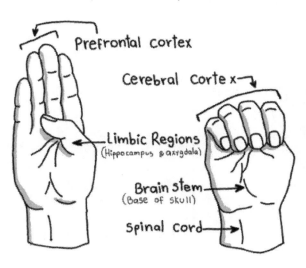

The model works like this: the "upstairs brain" is represented by the four fingers folded over the thumb. The four fingers represent the brain's cortex or outer bark, which is not fully developed in adolescents. The prefrontal cortex which is represented by the tips of the four fingers, is the area in the brain that controls analytic thinking, problem-solving, memory forming, time management, verbal communication, and free will. This area also helps us to be conscious and reason through life's situations. The knuckles, which are visible when the four fingers are bent over the thumb, represent the cerebral cortex (the outer part of the brain) which in this case, is important and supports cognitive control.

The "downstairs brain" is represented by the wrist and the palm of the hand. The lower palm can be thought of as the brain stem, which coordinates motor control and signals sent from the brain to the rest of the body. In this model, the wrist represents the spinal cord, which receives signals from the brainstem to control life-supporting autonomic functions of the peripheral nervous system among other things.

The thumb represents the limbic system, the area of the brain which is linked to emotions and reactive states like being scared or angry. Within the limbic system, we'll find the amygdala and hippocampus. The amygdala communicates closely with the hippocampus, which is responsible for memories and explains why we better remember things tied to emotions.

Remember when we talked about the "Panic Zone" in Chapter 2? The amygdala's key role is to determine how we respond to environmental threats and challenges by evaluating the emotional importance of sensory information and prompting an appropriate response. For example, does that bear pose a threat? Likely meeting a bear will be threatening. But physical danger is not the only threat the amygdala responds to. Fear of judgment, fear of saying the wrong thing, fear of being punished, fear of being called out, fear of failing, fear of rejection, and any other host of emotional experiences can also be perceived by your brain as a threat. All of these things can signal DANGER to the amygdala.

Let's look at what happens next.

When the amygdala perceives danger, emotions take control. We activate a state of fight, flight, freeze, or fawn. When this happens, Siegel calls this "flipping our lids." Imagine your hand responding to this temporary state by moving your four fingers straight up towards the sky. This shows you how the "upstairs brain" is no longer in control or connected to the "downstairs brain."

Teaching yourself and your teen the hand model of the brain can help create the vocabulary to understand what is driving the "irrational" behavior. When working with younger children, your role is to help your child "co-regulate" and bring the upstairs brain back into control. In working with your teen, you can partner with them, as long as you both clearly understand what is happening and have developed the language to talk about it. Unfortunately, oftentimes adults will unwittingly fuel the dysregulation by responding in ways the teenage brain continues to perceive as threatening. Hint: telling a child, a teen, or even your partner to "calm down" can cause the behavior to spiral because those words are adding yet another stressor.

If you haven't taken responsibility for learning how to manage your own emotional charges, you could also "flip your lid" and get pulled into the swirling dance of emotional dysregulation.

Use the hand model of the brain to help both you and your adolescent to become more mindful of helping the upstairs brain regain control.

The Biology of Fear

Fear is one of the most basic human emotions. From a survival standpoint, fear helps us to identify and recognize potential threats. As we've explored earlier, this powerful emotion has a direct line to our amygdala (part of our reptilian brain), kicking into action our fight, flight, freeze, or fawn responses. While fear is necessary to keep us safe, one of the big challenges of living in modern times (and in a time of COVID), we've become accustomed to perceiving more than just a bear on our path as a threat. Fears of the future, reputation, success, getting into the best college, paying bills, and potentially any other countless life situations can be fear-inducing. According to researchers, fear is killing us.

Put simply, fear always begins with a frightening stimulus and ends with our bodies preparing to protect themselves. Let's say you just noticed a large scary spider directly above your head right now (Did you look?) or your front door slams shut during the night. Or imagine something worse, perhaps encountering an intruder in your home, finding yourself face-to-face with their gun. Regardless of the situation, you could feel overwhelmed with fear, perhaps combined with anxiety, dread, or panic. Your digestive system slows, your pupils dilate, and your breathing speeds up. Your heart races like it could jump out of your chest, your breathing quickens and shallows, and most certainly your muscles tense up in anticipation for whatever is next...

All these reactions will involve separate parts of your brain, each instantaneously determining the appropriate responses. First, the thalamus processes the external information and signals in your body. Then, there are two potential paths by which the thalamus can choose to send information: through the downstairs brain or the upstairs brain.

The downstairs brain reacts to life-threatening situations like coming face-to-face with an intruder in your home. The thalamus alerts your amygdala and your fight, flight, freeze, or fawn response kicks in and takes over while the hypothalamus, which turns up your adrenal glands and rushes blood to your muscles to get you ready for action.

If the signal isn't life-threatening, the brain moves the response to the upstairs brain, which responds more rationally. Perhaps that large scary spider above your head gave you a fright, but you recognize you aren't in immediate danger, the amygdala alerts the prefrontal cortex to take over. This is why it's important to learn about these biological responses. The prefrontal cortex alerts the hippocampus, the brain's memory center, and immediately compares this current threat to past threats stored in your memory.

Your brain responds at break-neck speed, but this immediate response could have a long-term negative effect. With each fear response, an increased surge of hormones is sent to certain parts of the brain, primarily the amygdala and the hippocampus. One result of these increased hormones is storing the event in the hippocampus. According to researchers, once the fear pathways are experienced, the brain labels it as negative within your long-term memory along with storing details from that event such as the images, time of day, smells, feelings, etc.

When fear activation occurs, and we become hyper-aware and focused on a threat for extended periods of time, other events and memories can get fragmented or lost entirely. It may even affect our ability to form new long-term memories, and our brain may use our fear-tainted memories as confirmation that the world is indeed a fearful place. Then, whenever a similar fear stimulus shows up, the same array of emotions and memories from the first event resurface. That's what's known as *fear conditioning*.

Once fear conditioning occurs, sights, sounds, and other details similar to the original event can be transformed into new fear stimuli causing a triggered fear response. Seeing a photo of a large scary spider may trigger the fear you experienced when you initially saw the spider above your head, causing you to feel afraid without consciously knowing why.

Unfortunately, people can develop chronic fear. To them, the world becomes unsafe, and their memories will confirm that belief. A hyperactive amygdala can easily misread signals and misinterpret even the most innocent of situations. Experiencing heightened fear for a prolonged period of time can interrupt processes in our brains that allow us to regulate our emotions. Not having the ability to regulate ourselves, our thinking is impacted as is our decision-making ability, leaving us susceptible to intense emotional states and impulsive reactions.

Another byproduct of living in a constant state of fear is the overproduction of stress-related hormones. This causes the brain's natural levels of serotonin, dopamine, and oxytocin to be reduced. Without normal levels of these chemicals, we become susceptible to forming long-term mental health problems such as severe anxiety, depression, chronic stress disorders, and PTSD.

The process of overcoming *fear conditioning* is known as *fear extinction*. Fear extinction involves consciously creating new responses to fear-triggering situations. This includes making new and positive associations with the original fear, but this takes commitment to rewire and re-fire these auto-responses in the brain. When we are stuck in a chronic fear pattern, our ability to consciously choose another thought or emotional reaction diminishes.

Techniques like meditation, deep breathing, and focused thinking are all excellent tools to help break the fear cycle. You will also find tools in Chapter 9 to help you consciously reprogram your fears. However, if these techniques aren't enough, seeking help from a professional may be necessary.

The Power of Dopamine & Hyperrationality

For those who have never dived deep into learning about the biological side of human development, I recognize this chapter may be a bit overwhelming. But there is so much to consider as we try to form a comprehensive understanding of why our teens experience the world the way they do, why they make the decisions they do, and how this can affect their state of mental health. So, as always, I remind you here to take a deep breath and be patient with yourself as you start to integrate this knowledge into a greater comprehension of the adolescent brain.

As we explored teen myths in Chapter 3, we touched on the effects dopamine has on the adolescent brain and what hyper-rational thinking is. If you don't remember that section, please turn back to "Teens Are Impulsive" and reread that first myth – **it's important**. In this section, my goal is to help you expand your understanding of how these two elements affect your adolescence and provide you with a few tools and strategies to support your teen.

By now, you understand the brain is a collection of cells that communicate with one another using chemicals called neurotransmitters. Dopamine is the neurotransmitter that helps to control the brain's pleasure centers, creating a drive for reward. Baseline levels of dopamine are lowest during adolescence, at a time when they have the highest number of dopamine receptors. Dopamine releases can be an ecstasy-triggering response, especially appealing to adolescents who have a more developed limbic system, which is the key area responsible for processing emotional responses. Dopamine releases can give adolescents a powerful sensation of being alive and the desire to seek novelty to find these sensations. It can also prompt them to focus solely on the perceived rewards while failing to consider the potential risks.

As explained by Dr. Daniel Siegel, a better term for impulsivity would be "hyperrationality," or examining the facts of a situation and placing more "weight on the calculated benefits of an action than on the potential risks of that action." This is expressed by our adolescents' thinking in literal, concrete terms. In other words, teens have a hard time seeing the big picture and oftentimes completely miss the setting or context in which those decision-making considerations occur. Hyper-rational thinking is literally placing a lot of weight on the potential positive outcome and not much weight on potential negative consequences.

As a parent, please understand this is how all teens' brains are wired. They are participating in "logical-based reasoning" that has an inherent bias to automatically calculate the highest reward. I recognize reading that sentence might feel disempowering at this moment. With such literal thinking, what can we do to support our teens?

Here are my suggestions. Become a family that normalizes the following:

- **Remain in Partnership** – Partnership parenting means partnering with your adolescents to help them to feel empowered. Your choices and actions should make them feel like you are on their team and they can trust you. You are reading this book to support them, right? That's your role in the partnership. If needed, review Chapter 4.

- **Educate to Empower** – Help your teens to understand their own inner workings. Have conversations about their brain development and help them to understand the normal influence dopamine and hyperrationality have on their lives and their decisions. The more they know about their own biological development, the more empowered they will feel.

- **Do Not Shame or Judge** – Assure your teens there is no shame or judgment in being in the stage of life they are in. Celebrate adolescence together and all that is involved!

- **Do Not Take Things Personally** - This is for you, parents, I'll remind you of this tip over and over. Your teen's responses are (generally) NOT about you. If you find that their responses trigger you, that is your work. Cultivate awareness when you are taking things personally, getting triggered or applying expectations on your teen.

- **Do Not Punish, Instead Practice Natural Consequences** – Recognize there will be bad choices made by your teen. Commit now to not punishing them. Instead, through a culture of connection and dialogue around their mistakes, share with them your feelings and explore what natural consequences occur as a result of their choices.

- **Practice Naming Emotions** – Normalize naming emotions as they come up. As an example, model this practice and share your feelings. Print out a copy of the emotions wheel and tack it to the refrigerator. Naming what you are feeling in the heat of the moment has real biological benefits. Brain studies show that naming emotions activates the prefrontal cortex and calms emotions. Name it to tame it.

- **Use the Hand Model** – Teach the hand model of the brain and become a family that uses the hand model to demonstrate what is happening internally. The younger you normalize this practice with your children, the greater the benefits.

- **Wire Your Intuition With Your Heart** – Dr. Siegel recommends having adolescents put their hands on their chest and their stomach to become aware of the neural networks surrounding the intestines ("gut feeling") and the heart ("heartfelt feelings") and counter hyperrationality with intuition. Ask, "What do your heart and gut tell you about that plan?"

- **Adapt a Practice of Pausing** – Become a family that practices pausing before decisions are made. Normalize it as part of your family culture. Pausing has a biological effect on the developing adolescent brain. Pausing impulses affects regulatory fibers in the upstairs brain to create a mental space between impulse and action.

One of the best tips I always give to parents of teens is to start practicing taking a moment before deciding or acting and urge your teen to practice this as well. This habit can mean the difference between a positive and a negative outcome. Notice when your teen is acting without reflecting. Instead of judgment or criticism, encourage developing a practice of taking a pause first. The practice of pausing helps our teens to think about other options beyond the immediate dopamine-driven impulse pounding on their minds.

Pause Tool:

Write these 5 steps out and pin them somewhere everyone in your family can see them.

1. Declare it's time to take a pause.
2. Determine the emotion you are responding to.
3. Consider consequences.
4. Weigh harmful outcomes of potentially risky behaviors.
5. Seek more information or advice.

Resiliency & Plasticity

In Chapter 2, we briefly touched on the role plasticity plays as you develop deeper skills to support your teens. Here, we're going to focus on how neuroplasticity affects the adolescent brain.

As we previously explored, neuroplasticity is the brain's neural network's ability to change through growth and reorganization. This is true throughout the lifespan of every human, but through childhood and adolescence, the plasticity or ability to change is the highest. The process is driven by rewiring and firing sequences in neurons resulting in the formation of new cellular circuits. During different stages of human development, the brain is evolving and taking shape.

From the time of birth until about 3 years old, the brain has the most plasticity. This means that during this period, the brain is learning and synaptic firing is broadly developing. During adolescence, the brain will start to connect these synapses in ways to provide greater context to their life. Because of this, a wide variety of ideas, thoughts, and concepts are being connected and meaning is given (that may or may not actually be true).

In the adolescent brain, new cells are constantly being produced and their interconnectivity is sculpted during the process of synaptic pruning as we discussed earlier. Synaptic connections are being formed which help us to reason, plan, problem-solve, and determine right from wrong.

An example of how this sequence might look in real life is:

- Doing crazy things with my friends gives me attention
- Attention gives me a sense of approval
- Approval makes me feel good
- I feel good when I'm crazy

Adolescence is a time when the brain is striving to make meaning. In normal times, teens experience high levels of activation of the amygdala in the subcortical region of the brain from increased environmental stressors and task demands, heightened emotional experiences, and peer pressure. The recent societal changes as a result of the COVID-19 pandemic have likely accelerated these influences and added heightened fear stimuli, unpredicted changes, and numerous messages of uncertainty, all of which can contribute to sensory overload. Thus, as a result of the times we are living, the rewiring of the adolescent brain can be susceptible to negative belief patterns that increase the burden of stress, grief, anxiety, and fear.

In order to best support your teens, you must understand that changes occurring in your teen's neural networks during adolescence can influence the way they experience the world into adulthood. Neuroplasticity can influence their wiring either positively or negatively, and you can make a difference in which has the greatest influence. Here are some important tools you can use to facilitate greater mental health in your adolescent:

- Encourage listening to their own emotional spark in order to keep their passions active.

- Encourage strong relationships strong within their social networks and support social engagement with their peers.
- Encourage novelty and facilitate trying new things.
- Encourage mind expansion and challenges through creative exploration.
- Encourage compassion and practice empathy.

Self-Regulation

Parents, is it not tempting to label our teen's challenging behaviors as rebellious, oppositional, defiant, manipulative, or attention-seeking? Actually, those behaviors oftentimes are not intentional; they can be a result of not being able to handle the big emotions (remember the activated limbic system?). When adolescents feel overwhelmed, their feelings may get the best of them, preventing them from being able to self-regulate.

Simply put, self-regulation is the ability to remain calm, cope with the big emotions, adapt, and respond appropriately to the current environment. It's also the individual's ability to influence or control their own impulses, which requires some element of emotional intelligence. Is this a skill you've cultivated in your own life? If not, this section will support both you and your teen.

Let's use the analogy of the upstairs and downstairs brain again in order to understand which areas contribute to self-regulation.

When teens feel safe and relaxed, the upstairs brain (the prefrontal cortex) is mostly leading. The dominant effects are self-awareness and self-control. This is also the part of the brain that allows us to pause before action, and this takes practice. Practicing pausing helps us to activate the upstairs brain, thus helping us to self-regulate.

As we've explored, the upstairs brain takes time to fully develop. This means that teens biologically have greater difficulty with self-regulation than adults, but as they move through their adolescents, they develop greater skills, allowing them to more easily adapt and calm.

Remember when your teen was a young child? Big emotions could have easily propelled your child into a full-blown meltdown, making it difficult for them to cope with and adapt to change. The ability to calm themselves or regulate when feeling overwhelmed becomes easier over time as their upstairs brain develops but bringing awareness to the biological stages of growth can bring greater understanding and compassion for your teen and prompt your teen to start applying self-compassion to themselves.

The downstairs brain includes the limbic system, which controls our emotion and stress responses (fight, flight, freeze, and fawn). When our downstairs brain senses danger, it prompts us straight into the action. This survival instinct sends adrenaline pumping through our bodies, which can be the difference between life or death in a dangerous situation. As we know, a problem can arise when our downstairs brain wrongly interprets everyday stress as a danger. The many teens I've worked with since the beginning of the pandemic have expressed a heightened sense of danger in what would have previously been perceived as normal everyday activities. When teens are challenged to meet the changing demands of their environment, their strong emotional responses can trigger their fight, flight, freeze, or fawn response automatically. Unfortunately, this ongoing stimulus prompted by the pandemic can lead to a combination of social, emotional, and behavioral challenges.

Normally as teens move through their adolescence, you should be able to notice their ability to better manage thoughts, emotions, and behaviors. Research shows that when teens learn and practice self-regulation skills, they are forming new neural pathways (neuroplasticity) that increase their ability to manage stress. As the parent, you can encourage, support, and acknowledge these natural skills as they develop in your teen:

- Practice pausing
- Choosing to stay calm
- Making responsible, future-focused choices
- Focusing and applying self-discipline techniques to avoid distraction
- Working towards goals

- Adapting to changes in the environment
- Cooperating and collaborating

As we know, adolescents (and to be fair, adults too) do not always handle the big emotions elegantly. As a result, teens may appear anxious, irritable, impulsive, destructive, or aggressive. To make matters more difficult for parents, sometimes teens internalize overwhelming frustration in ways we cannot see. Developing a culture of emotional intelligence in your family is crucial.

One of the ways in which self-regulation contributes to well-being is through emotional intelligence. Mayer and Salovey best summarized emotional intelligence as "the ability to perceive emotions, to access and generate emotions so as to assist thought, to understand emotions and emotional knowledge, and to reflectively regulate emotions so as to promote emotional and intellectual growth."

According to emotional intelligence expert Daniel Goleman, there are five components of emotional intelligence:

1. Self-awareness
2. Self-regulation
3. Internal motivation
4. Empathy
5. Social skills

Self-regulation and emotional intelligence function hand in hand. Imagine your teen developing high levels of self-awareness, intrinsic motivation, empathy, and social skills. Those who cultivate those skills will also develop control over their own impulses and emotions. This supports your teen's overall well-being.

In the midst of teens' responses, whether it's "attitude," snappy comebacks, the eye rolls, or simply ignoring you, your challenge is to self-regulate despite what they are doing. When we are calm, we can better respond with compassion and patience towards our teens. This is clearly our work and our responsibility within the partnership paradigm.

Children mirror the stress and emotional responses of the adults around them. If they are dysregulated, offer a gentle touch, empathize, and validate their feelings. Recognize that adolescents need time and support to learn and practice regulation skills. More importantly, recognize they won't always get it right. Regardless, it is imperative you model self-regulation by remaining calm.

IF **EMOTIONS** COULD TALK

SADNESS might be telling me I need TO CRY

LONELINESS might be telling me I need CONNECTION

SHAME might be telling me I need SELF-COMPASSION

RESENTMENT might be telling me I need TO FORGIVE

EMPTINESS might be telling me I need TO DO SOMETHING CREATIVE

ANGER might be telling me I need TO CHECK-IN WITH MY BOUNDARIES

ANXIETY might be telling me I need TO BREATHE

STRESS might be telling me I need TO TAKE IT ONE STEP AT A TIME

Creating safe spaces to talk about and normalize feelings and assuring your teens there will never be punishment can help your adolescence develop important self-regulation skills. Choosing connection over coercion (remember Chapter 4?) is crucial as punishment will likely frustrate your teens more, leading to feelings of shame and failure, thus increasing the challenges of self-regulation.

Self-regulation involves developing a set of skills that help us to manage our big emotions and think before we act. As the parent, here are some ways you can support your teen's self-regulation skills:

- Manage your own stress.
- Model your own self-regulation.
- Commit to supporting your adolescents' self-regulation, not with the intent to control their behavior, but to support developing new skills.
- Do not try to reason with your teen while they are dysregulated. Remember, the lower brain is in control.
- Normalize dialogue around emotions and promote emotional intelligence in your family.
- Prepare yourself for the challenge and develop realistic expectations.
- Expect setbacks; they're part of the process.
- Be supportive and encouraging.
- Reduce unnecessary demands.
- Provide consistency. In some cases, predictability helps to decrease stress.
- Collaborate and make learning about self-regulation enjoyable.
- Provide your teen-specific feedback.
- Focus on effort over results.

Cultivating skills for self-regulation in adolescents is linked to positive outcomes, which support well-being for life. In the 2016 study "Emotion Regulation Strategies and Psychosocial Well-being in Adolescence," researchers showed that adolescents who regularly engaged in self-regulatory behavior reported greater well-being than their peers. The benefits include enhanced life satisfaction, perceived social support, and overall positivity. From the same study, the adolescents who suppressed their feelings, instead of addressing them head-on, experienced a lower sense of well-being, including heightened loneliness, more bad feelings, and worse overall psychological health.

Here are some exercises you can try with yourself and with your teen to practice self-regulation.

Box Breathing

Box breathing is one of my favorite techniques used to regulate the nervous system. This technique has been used in a variety of settings, from doctors' and therapists' offices to yoga studios and meditation centers. Even Navy SEALs are trained to use box breathing to stay calm and improve their concentration in extremely tense situations.

The technique is simple, and as the name suggests, it entails breathing in a pattern symbolized by a box.

> Step 1: Inhale through the nose to a slow count of four, completely filling your lungs with air.

> Step 2: Hold your breath, keeping the air in your lungs for the same time, a count of four.

> Step 3: Exhale through your mouth to the same pace of a count of four, completely emptying out your lungs.

> Step 4: With your lungs in an empty state, count to four using the same pace as above.

> Step 5: Repeat the sequence one through four for a duration of five minutes.

Mindfulness

Another powerful practice for self-regulation is mindfulness. In the Suggested Reading section, I've listed many titles on this subject, my favorite in the bunch being *Growing Up Mindful: Essential Practices to Help Children, Teens, and Families Find Balance, Calm, and Resilience* by Christopher Willard.

Basically, mindfulness is defined as the conscious effort to maintain moment-to-moment awareness of one's internal worlds, including our thoughts and feelings while maintaining an awareness of the outer world concurrently. Mindfulness is often thought of as a type of meditation in which you focus on being intensely aware of what you're sensing and feeling in the moment, without interpretation or judgment. Practicing mindfulness involves breathing methods, guided imagery, and other practices to relax the body and mind and help reduce stress. Mindfulness supports self-regulation and, in combination, is a powerful duo in pursuit of well-being.

I would argue becoming conscious of your own thoughts, feelings, and behavior is the foundation of self-regulation. Without it, there is no ability to reflect or choose a different path.

Through practicing mindfulness, you can become actively aware of your own thoughts and feelings and promote conscious decisions about how to behave instead of simply going along with whatever your feelings tell you.

Body Scan

One of my favorite mindfulness activities to facilitate is the mindful meditation practice of the body scan. You can facilitate this exercise with your teen or teach them how to do it themselves. The body scan directs your focused attention on the sensations happening from within your body. Systematically starting at your toes, you focus attention from the inside out and work your way up to the crown of your head, feeling sensations without judgment.

One of my favorite ways to practice this technique is to focus my attention on each body part by closing my eyes and imagining a warm, yellow glow surrounding each area. If I feel any pain, I allow the warm, yellow glow to melt away any tension in the area. This practice is very relaxing and a great way to slow the momentum of your thoughts.

Dr. Daniel Siegel has a tool he developed called the Wheel of Awareness practice, which I highly recommend. This tool provides the basis for a reflective practice, which helps you direct your attention and improve your ability to focus on the individual aspects of your internal and external worlds, which are key components of a healthy mind. You can find out more about this tool by checking out the chart and accessing the recordings of the guided meditations here: https://drdansiegel.com/wheel-of-awareness/

The Lion Mind Metaphor

The metaphor of the Lion Mind, as a way to describe mindfulness, comes from David Guy and Larry Rosenberg's book *Breath by Breath: The Liberating Practice of Insight Meditation.* This metaphor has also been used by Sam Himelstein, Ph.D., founder and CEO of the Center for Adolescent Studies, in his practice facilitating mindfulness and emotional intelligence skills with incarcerated and marginalized youth.

The metaphor is simple and only takes a moment to present. Hold up a pen and ask your teen to imagine you are holding a bone. Ask them to imagine you are now standing in front of a sitting dog, and you start to slowly move the bone from left to right in front of the dog's face. Ask your teen to imagine the dog's head moving left to right as you wave this bone. Then, imagine you toss the bone a few feet away. Ask, "What will the dog do?"

Himelstein explains the response he usually gets is the dog will chase the bone.

Now, ask your teen to imagine you are now standing in front of a lion. Imagine you are waving the bone in the lion's face from side to side and then tossing it a few yards away. Ask your teen once again, "What will the lion do?

More than likely, your teen will conclude the lion will eat you. True. The fact is the lion just might eat you in that situation.

Invite your teen to recognize there is a fundamental difference between the mind of the dog and the mind of the lion. The dog has tunnel vision and can't really see beyond the bone. In the case of the dog, the metaphor is simple. If one controls the bone, one controls the dog's reality.

Now, examine the situation with the lion, which of course is fundamentally different. The lion too sits upright. However, as you wave the bone, the lion's eyes will be looking beyond the bone and directly at you. The lion understands the bone is just a small piece of a larger reality and therefore has much more autonomy. In reality, the lion has many choices, but the nature of the lion won't be like that of the dog, a slave to the thrown bone. The lion will sit, consider, and look at the whole situation. After all that, the likely choice the lion may make is to pounce on you and rip you into shreds, so clearly do not try this exercise in real life.

In this metaphor, the bone represents our experiences, emotions, perceptions, situations, or environments. Ask your teen to identify some of the bones they have recently experienced. An example may be that bone represented "worry" yesterday. Ask your teen which mind they employed when interacting with that bone. Were they extremely anxious? Did they get caught up in chasing the bones of worrying thoughts? Ask your teen to consider if they got caught up in their own story of the bone. Ask them to identify the thoughts, images, sensations, and emotions that were the bone. Now, ask your teen to imagine they are sitting with autonomy, embodying the spirit of the lion. What does that feel or look like?

By remembering the image of the lion sitting there, being present and non-reactive, we remind ourselves of the state of mind we are trying to cultivate through mindfulness. We are not necessarily relaxed, but we are present with the nonreactive and nonjudgmental attitude of a lion. By cultivating the ability to be mindful, we can face whatever bones get thrown our way.

Reticular Activating System

Motivational speakers and self-help gurus like Anthony Robbins and Mel Robbins (not related) both have stumbled upon the science behind reprogramming your experiences, meeting goals, and changing your mindset. I personally am a huge fan of Mel Robbins' two books *The 5 Second Rule* and *The High 5 Habit*. The guiding science behind both books is our ability to tap into the reticular activating system.

The reticular activating system (RAS) is a bundle of nerves located at the brainstem whose job is to help the brain sort out the two-billion bits of information received every second and determine what is important to us. The RAS acts as a filter that processes sensory input gathered through our five senses and sifts through the responding conscious and subconscious thoughts. This busy filter is at work 24/7 and keeps us from becoming overwhelmed by the mass amount of information our brains are constantly processing.

Did you know?
You can "rewire" your brain to
be happy by simply recalling
3 things you're grateful for
every day for 21 days.

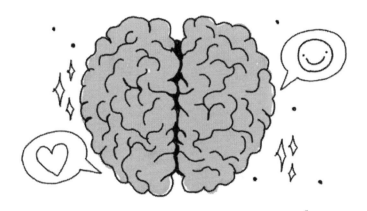

Essentially, the RAS acts as the brain's gatekeeper, deciding what we consciously give our attention to. Our core beliefs help the RAS sift through and prioritize which information, stimulus, or input is perceived by the conscious thinking mind. The RAS is biased, oftentimes overlooking neutral and even positive occurrences to confirm the beliefs the brain habitually practices (either consciously or subconsciously). Confirmation bias originates from the RAS creating filters that agree with our belief systems.

So, if you constantly feel like you're a horrible parent, guess what? Your reticular activating system will go through your day and filter out any experiences or messages contrary to that belief. It will also bring into focus every single piece of evidence confirming that negative belief you have about yourself.

Does this sound like you are fighting an uphill battle? Does it feel impossible to exit this continuous loop? The good news is you are not doomed. Just as we explored in the section about neuroplasticity, we can change and reprogram our minds. It just takes some conscious effort.

The 30-30-30 Tool

I have created a tool I call 30-30-30. As with all the tools in this book, I suggest you try this tool yourself before trying to facilitate this tool with your adolescent. The tool requires a thirty-day commitment to shift the dominant programming present in your reticular activating system. The 30-30-30 tool requires a little planning, but over the duration of the next thirty days, you will need to commit to two thirty-second intervals per day when you are focused. That's it. Essentially just one minute a day, the same time each day, in order for you to get the maximum benefit. Ready? Let's get started.

> **Step 1: Choose a limiting belief** or a negative thought you are committing to focusing on for this month.
>
> Many of us have negative beliefs stacked upon each other. Without having experience in practicing self-inquiry, the top belief may be the easiest to access. Let's start there. For those who have uncovered your deeper core wounds, dig right in with one of those. There is often a domino effect as you start to reprogram the core wounds, and the beliefs stacked on top of that core wound tend to disappear.
>
> **Step 2: Choose the reality you want.** Like we did with Byron Katie's *The Work* in Chapter 4, we need to find a way to turn around the limiting belief you just chose. Search for the most powerful way to rephrase the negative belief to make it a positive aspiration. Feel free to use your imagination, reach high, make it big, and unbelievable. Go big or go home, right?
>
> For example, if we are using the thought, "I'm a bad parent," you can choose to reprogram that belief with the opposite thought, "I am a great parent," "I'm the world's best mom," or "I have the most

amazing, strong, connected relationships with my kids." Make it your own, make it big, make it extraordinary.

Step 3: Write out what that statement means to you. Activate your imagination and write out what that reality means. If you need to, imagine a world of fantasy or put another person in your place to create the story. Do whatever you need to do to narrate the most innovative positive description of that statement possible. Write about the scene, the colors, the interactions, the sights, the smells, the people, the dialogue, the feelings, and anything else you can think of! Give yourself permission to go fantastic, full-blown fantasy.

Use the notes section in the back of this book if you don't have a notebook handy.

Step 4: Find a time and commit to it. Select a time, the exact same time of the day, for the next thirty days to activate the 30-30-30 Tool. The actual time you are committing to is two thirty-second sessions, equaling a total of one minute. That's it! One minute each day, at the same time of the day, to activate this tool. Make a promise to yourself now and keep it. The best time I've found for me is committing to the morning before I get out of bed, but some of the teens I work with prefer nighttime before they go to sleep. You will need to have a phone or a timer accessible.

Step 5: Get ready. Start!

Part 1: Set your timer for 30 seconds. For 30 seconds, visualize, think, and fantasize about the scenes you described with your new "I statement." If you need to for the first couple of days, you can read what you wrote. See the scene in your mind. Watch the scene play out of you being "the world's best mom." Visualize every detail you can see: your face, your kids' faces, the interactions, the connections. As you move through the thirty days, the scene may organically progress, morph, and expand. But if you need to keep seeing the same scene over and over, that works too. Don't force anything, just be present and use your mind's eye to visualize this new chosen reality. Thirty seconds go fast, so be wholly committed to the process for that duration of time.

Part 2: Reset the timer for a second 30-second interval. This time, spend the next thirty seconds feeling the emotions you felt from witnessing the scenes you just saw in your mind's eye. Recognize the joy, the love, the gratitude, and the presence you feel. Name the emotions in your mind as they come up. Notice how your heart feels, how energy moves through your body, the awareness of where emotions radiate in the different areas of yourself, and if there are any other sensations you are aware of. Spend this 30-second period deeply feeling.

Bonus: If you have time, journal your experiences. The added focus and attention will help reset your RAS, but the 30-30-30 Tool works fine without.

Step 6: Repeat for 30 days. You've made your commitment. Now, repeat the same thing for thirty days. Mark it on your calendar. If you need to, have an alarm that goes off to remind you it's time to activate your 30-30-30 Tool.

The 30-30-30 Tool reprograms you. The new positive belief becomes the dominant and activated thought. The old belief is no longer in the foreground. As a result of using this tool, your brain will start encoding the belief as if it is a real memory. The thirty seconds of emotional charge around the new thought anchors the new thought in your mind. Encoded memories change the filter active in your reticular activating system, and the confirmation bias will be focused on your new programmed thought.

Based on scientific research, the more you visualize yourself in new situations, the more your mind helps you to develop the skills, see the opportunities, and access the right things to say. As you practice seeing and feeling the new thought, your brain is building new neural connections and creating new beliefs.

Cognitive Development Throughout Adolescence

All the tools I present in this book are designed to expand your understanding, support your connection, and contribute to the greater overall mental health of yourself and your teen. Sometimes reading a list of developmental qualities helps us in our parenting to normalize some of the perceived madness we may be living. The natural internal and biological development adolescents are experiencing affects everyone in the family.

This amazing list published by Stanford Children's Health will help you to understand the stages of cognitive development taking place during adolescence and perhaps assist you in being a little more patient. The three stages are: Early Adolescence, Middle Adolescence, and Late Adolescence. Hopefully, this list below will give you an idea of what to expect in your teen's normal cognitive growth through the years.

Early Adolescence (Roughly Ages 12-15)
- Uses more complex thinking focused on personal decision-making
- Begins to show the use of formal logical operations in project work
- Begins to question authority and society's standards
- Begins to form and speak his or her own thoughts and views on many topics. You may hear your teen talk about which sports or groups he or she prefers, what kinds of personal appearance is attractive, and what parental rules should be changed.

Middle Adolescence (Roughly Ages 16-19)
- Has some experience in using more complex thinking processes
- Expands thinking to include more philosophical and futuristic concerns
- Often questions more extensively
- Often analyzes more extensively
- Thinks about and begins to form his or her own code of ethics
- Thinks about different possibilities and begins to develop their own identity
- Thinks about and begins to systematically consider possible future goals (for example, What do I want?)

- Thinks about and begins to make his or her own plans
- Begins to think long term
- Uses systematic thinking and begins to influence relationships with others

Late Adolescence (Roughly Ages 20-25)
- Uses complex thinking to focus on less self-centered concepts and personal decision-making
- Has increased thoughts about more global concepts, such as justice, history, politics, and patriotism
- Often develops idealistic views on specific topics or concerns
- May debate and develop intolerance of opposing views
- Begins to focus thinking on making career decisions
- Begins to focus thinking on their emerging role in adult society

One of the ways you can integrate this knowledge into supporting healthy cognitive growth is to encourage your teen to share their opinions on a wide variety of topics, issues, and current events. Listen without judgment and encourage your teen to share their ideas and thoughts with you. Supporting your teen to think independently helps them to develop their own ideas about things. Create safe spaces for differing opinions and practice regulating your nervous systems when disagreements occur. Support your teen to think about and set goals. Acknowledge your teen for well-thought-out decisions. Create a culture of support, helping your teen to re-evaluate poorly made decisions.

Chapter 7: Red Flags

I am certain you are reading this book because you deeply wish for your teen to be healthy, happy, and thrive in life. When someone you love is struggling, hurting, sad, or confused, it's natural to be concerned. It can be difficult to know when to step in or when these changes are a natural part of growing up.

Everyone struggles at different times in their lives. We all experience stress, sadness, and a variety of emotions. Each and every person reacts to stressors in different ways. What may be a healthy form of expression for one person could be a warning sign for another person. As a parent, it's hard to know exactly when you should be concerned.

As you know, I am not a therapist, psychologist, or a doctor. This chapter is dedicated to helping you understand what red flags are and recognize certain patterns or behaviors that might be of concern in your adolescent's life. If there is ever any question, I urge you to seek the support of a professional.

Unfortunately, there is no one-size-fits-all guide to rely on. It's never as simple as identifying a specific symptom or behavior as an automatic sign of mental or emotional distress. Instead, the best advice is to look for changes in behavior. All the signs or symptoms mentioned below will require a combination of a parent's natural instinct and conscious thought to determine just how serious the issues may be.

Think about your teen's "normal." Then, look at any changes from their baseline and ask yourself, "Is my teen acting differently than I would normally expect?" Always look for patterns or escalating behaviors.

For parents, this is hard work. You must rely on your intuition and objectivity as you observe what is going on with your teen. Equally, you must be able to separate your perception from your own belief system and personal triggers. Remember, your teen is an autonomous being, independent of you, with their own standards, values, and interests. It is up to you to be objective and make sure the lens you are observing their behaviors through isn't clouded by your judgment or expectations. Again, this is hard work for us as parents.

Also recognize that within the Western world, we are conditioned to believe experiencing any level of anxiety or depression could be dangerous. In actuality, these experiences, if not chronic, are not intrinsically bad, just uncomfortable. As we know, when most people enter the space of being uncomfortable, they have the impulse to change, fix, or solve the situation instead of enjoying the discomfort. However, it's vital to be able to distinguish the difference between being in the stretch zone (as defined in Chapter 2) and a red flag.

Most red flags will fall into one or more of these four categories:

- Physical functioning - Is your teen sleeping too much or not enough? Have their eating patterns changed? Have their energy patterns altered from their baseline normal? Were they someone who was typically energetic, and now they are acting lethargic? Has your teen not gotten out of bed for days?

- Emotional functioning - Is your teen more irritable? Are they sad or gloomy about their life? Is your teen more easily frustrated than normal? Are they crying more often? Is your teen talking about no longer having the will to live?

- Cognitive functioning - Are there changes in the way your teen is interpreting or internalizing events around them? Are they having a more difficult time being rational about changes beyond their control? Is your teen responding with illogical responses to things that they had normally been able to handle?

- Behavioral functioning - Has your teen made radical changes in their friends, interests, or appearance? Has your teen stopped caring about the things they used to be interested in? Has your teen participated in self-harm or expressed the desire to hurt others?

Change in Sleep Patterns

I'm surprised this is the first opportunity I've had to mention adolescent's sleep patterns.

As a parent of a teen, you have likely already witnessed a change in their natural sleep schedule, as most teens prefer to stay up later and sleep in later. Our circadian rhythms are the biological and psychological processes that follow the cycle of our 24-hour internal clock. The biological changes taking place in an adolescent's body affect their internal clock, delaying the time they start feeling sleepy and the time they would naturally arise. Teens naturally stay up later at night and sleep later during the day if they are not affected by enforced schedules, such as those dictated by school.

Being sleepy throughout the day is a common trait of an adolescent. But if they are sleeping drastically more or less for several weeks, it could be a sign of issues including depression, anxiety, insomnia, or substance abuse.

Loss of Interest in Favorite Activities

As we touched on in Chapters 3 and 6, the adolescent brain is actively remodeling itself. Some of the experiences, thoughts, memories, emotions, and information are being dropped as the young mind determines what is important to them and what is not. Some interests may no longer be of interest to your developing teen as the pruning process continues.

For example, it's normal for a teen to switch their passion from soccer to theater. But when you notice your teen becoming more withdrawn or start making radical and abrupt changes to their passions, it could be an indication of several issues including depression, anxiety, bipolar disorder, bullying, or undiagnosed ADD.

Anger Issues

Anger is experienced by everyone from time to time. As we've explored throughout this book, teens often perceive things very differently than adults do. Because of the heightened emotional processing and hyper-rationalization, adolescents' thinking may be distorted at times. Keep a mindful eye when your teens use hyperrational thinking to justify angry behavior. This kind of faulty thinking is not something adolescents engage in intentionally, rather they are subject to automatic thinking. They might say, "It's not my fault; the world sucks!" or "Someone stole my backpack. Everyone is out to get me!" or "My boss hates me. Why should I do what he says anyway?"

If your teen experiences really strong impulses and doesn't have the tools to manage or cope, it may become a difficult situation for the whole family. However, when explosive anger turns into a violent rage, this definitely is a red flag. You will likely need support to manage the situation.

Depression

In its most basic form, depression is a mood disorder that causes a persistent feeling of sadness. Everyone feels the sensation of depression from time to time over their lifetime, but I distinguish this from the major depressive disorder called clinical depression, which is sometimes caused by a chemical imbalance in the brain. Clinical depression affects how a person thinks, feels, and behaves and usually leads to a variety of emotional and physical challenges.

In order to determine if this is indeed a red flag or a normal feeling of the blues, you must look objectively at your adolescent's behavior, state of mind, and the duration of the feeling of sadness. Oftentimes, depression is a consequence of chronic hyper-focusing on an event, a circumstance, or series of events that have already occurred. Commonly, a person creates an absolute meaning, a limiting belief, about one's identity as a result of feeling helpless. You can help your teen explore feelings of sadness through the tools in Chapter 9.

In Eckhart Tolle's book *The Power of Now*, Tolle explains the process of emotional imprinting, which he calls the pain body, as it takes over the rational mind and perpetuates compulsive negative thinking to keep the pain alive. Much like the reticular activating system, once your mind has practiced a dominant thought for a period of time, it becomes all you notice and experience.

Unpacking the thoughts and beliefs under the emotional response helps to dismantle the power of the pain body. However, keep in mind chronic bouts of depression may require professional support.

Suicide Ideation

Suicide ideation is a broad term used to describe a wide range of thoughts, contemplations, wishes, and preoccupations with death and/or suicide. Unfortunately, there is no universally accepted definition of "suicide ideation," which leads to ongoing challenges for parents. It may become more challenging for parents to know what their teens are thinking and feeling, especially if their teen has withdrawn from the family during adolescence.

In this section, I'll unpack the important factors to look for that may be indications of a teen being at risk for suicide. The key to distinguishing a normal bad day from a risk of suicide may be found in noticing patterns or prolonged emotional states.

Research shows that 9 in 10 teens who end up taking their own lives meet the criteria for a diagnosis of a mental health disorder such as depression or anxiety. People who are suffering from depression often retreat into themselves but may be secretly crying out for help. Oftentimes, a person with suicide ideation feels shame around their thoughts and may be embarrassed to reveal their deep sadness to their parents.

Many teens who have suicidal thoughts reveal their distressed state of mind through their behaviors. As parents, we need to watch out for them. Poor communication between parents and their teens is a common trait within many families who have been affected by suicide. Studies show that often three or more of the following issues present at once as contributing factors to suicide ideation:

- Major loss (relationship breakups or death)
- Peer or social pressure
- Access to weapons
- Public humiliation
- Bullying
- Clinical depression
- Anxiety disorder
- Panic attacks
- Severe chronic pain
- Chronic medical condition
- No impulse control
- Drug or alcohol abuse
- Self-harm
- Bouts of aggressiveness
- Talking about suicide or threatening suicide
- Family history of suicide

Often, children who attempt suicide had been telling their parents repeatedly that they intended to kill themselves. Here are some examples of statements to watch out for:

"Nothing matters."
"I wonder how many people would come to my funeral."
"Sometimes I wish I could just go to sleep forever."
"The world would be better off without me."
"You won't have to worry about me much longer."

Please don't shrug off these comments or threats of suicide as typical teenage melodrama. Any of these statements could be a red flag warning, which should demand your immediate attention and action. If your instinct tells you your teen might be a danger to themself, listen to your instincts.

Anxiety

A classic definition of anxiety is excessive thinking about the future and what could happen. We all experience anxiety. It is natural to worry about any number of things that may or may not happen. Normal anxiety is not necessarily a red flag, but there are few things you must take notice of before it becomes an anxiety disorder.

There are a variety of anxiety disorders such as panic disorders, social anxiety, obsessive-compulsive disorders, phobias, and generalized anxiety disorders to name a few. All anxiety disorders have one predominant feature characterized by significant and uncontrollable feelings of anxiousness, worry, and fear, causing normal functioning to be significantly impaired. If you notice a pattern of these characteristics or prolonged anxiousness, this is a red flag. Untreated anxiety disorders can result in full-blown panic attacks and other physical manifestations that can lead to long-term issues.

How do we help our teens manage normal anxiety in an uncertain world? Use the tools we will discuss in Chapter 9 to help with processing worries and fears in a healthy way. Use tools like the emotion wheel to uncover each of the emotions they may be feeling and practice and normalize by giving them a name. You can use trigger logs to track when these emotions come up and notice the common thread behind these triggers. Also, Byron Katie's *The Work* can provide a tool to shift fears into manageable thoughts.

Eating Disorders

Eating disorders are life-or-death challenges. Especially for girls, disorders like anorexia and bulimia are getting a lot of attention in light of social media perpetuating an impossible definition of beauty and an "ideal" body image. Both anorexia and bulimia usually are combined with some sort of body dysmorphia, which is characterized by the obsessive idea that some aspect of one's body part or appearance is severely flawed. This thought usually causes a lot of internal shame and self-loathing.

Anorexia nervosa is a serious eating disorder. Individuals with anorexia do not eat enough calories and have an intense fear of being or becoming fat. Although the term anorexia nervosa means "no appetite caused by nervousness," most people with anorexia do feel hunger but go to extreme lengths to curb it, often to the point of starvation. At times, this disorder can be a response to the feeling of a lack of control over one's life with severe consequences. Bulimia nervosa is an eating disorder characterized by binge eating, followed by purging and often feeling plagued with concerns over body shape and weight.

One of the red flags to look out for in your teen is sudden changes in eating habits like becoming a picky eater or rejecting their old favorite foods. A day or two might be okay, but anything beyond that represents a shift in mental attitude and is not indicative of a simple loss in appetite. Notice the patterns.

Another sign may be a sudden rise in food intake. Sudden trips to the bathroom, particularly right after eating, can be an important sign to keep an eye on. Watch out for this pattern, especially if the big meal is followed by your teen eating very little or nothing for several meals before and/or after. This is a classic sign of bulimia. Individuals with bulimia respond to the binging by purging the body of food intake in a very harmful way, such as induced vomiting or the use of laxatives.

Having a healthy or weight-conscious teen is not necessarily a red flag but notice when their attitude changes from concern to obsession and take it as an acute warning sign. If your teen breaks into tears after stepping onto the scale for the nineteenth time today, this can be an indicator there is a developing problem.

Also, keep a watchful eye for an unhealthy obsession with exercise, particularly exercises focusing on calorie-burning, high-impact aerobics. Good health, body toning, and strength training can all be good for a growing body, but if your teen slavishly does the same exercise over and over just to burn fat, that can be a red flag.

Some of the physical signs to notice vitamin or protein deficiencies caused by eating disorders are problems reflected in unhealthy-looking skin, a noticeable decline in the quality of their hair or fingernails, and possibly enamel erosion on their teeth or tooth decay.

Often, parents find it difficult to distinguish the difference between changing food preferences and the beginnings of an eating disorder. Please be diligent in noticing patterns of change that will send up a red flag. If your teen requires intervention, you may encounter heated denials and objections, so make sure you have accurately recorded all the signs and incidents.

If you suspect your teen may be suffering from an eating disorder, you cannot simply pretend this is just a phase. Many adolescents go to great lengths to hide their disorder, and many can be very cunning in their attempts to keep the signs a secret. As a parent, you need to be very smart about recognizing the early signs of eating disorders.

Not all eating disorders are set into motion through body dysmorphia though. A couple of years ago, I worked with a younger teen who had a severe "push and pull" relationship with her mother. The teen internalized the lack of control in her life by developing an unhealthy relationship with food. Her experience with an overbearing mother caused her to assert some control over herself by limiting her food intake. From an early age, she developed an emotional response to food, almost all food making her gag.

In this case, this teen became dangerously unhealthy both physically and mentally. I advocated for her personally and helped to convince her mother she should admit her daughter into a treatment center. The mother objected for many months because she felt she could control or force her daughter to eat, which escalated in her disorder transforming from anorexia into bulimia. Finally, the teen was admitted. In the teen's mind, she finally gained some control over her life but recognized there was a long road of recovery ahead of her.

Some of the effects of prolonged eating disorders can be seen with menstrual or reproductive irregularities, kidney disease, osteoporosis, and even heart problems. Even when the disease is "cured," it can still generate health problems throughout their life.

Eating disorders almost always require professional assistance or intervention. Screaming at your teen or trying to control their behavior won't prompt them to stop having an eating disorder. Professional intervention can help your teen to address the hidden emotional issues that triggered the disorder in the first place.

Self-Harm

Self-harm is when a person intentionally injures their own body. Some of the common expressions of self-harm are cuts to arms, legs, or torso, frequent pulling of hair and eyelashes, or burns on the skin. These are all red flags to look for. Teens who self-harm often go to great lengths to hide their behavior, their wounds, or their scars, so you need to be diligent with your observations. If you suspect your adolescent is self-harming, please connect and confront your teen immediately.

Some of the reasons adolescents may self-harm include:

- An expression of emotional distress
- A coping mechanism
- Relief from emotional pain
- Releasing overwhelming tension
- Responding to intrusive thoughts
- An attempt to assert control
- A form of self-punishment
- Low self-esteem or self-loathing
- A cry for help

Self-harm can be linked to current stressors or past stressors alike. One of the teens I recently worked with explained the reason they self-harm is that they don't feel any control of their outer world, and this was exacerbated by COVID restrictions. But their self-harm isn't entirely about asserting control over their outer-world situation; it was a way to control the overwhelm they were feeling. They explained self-harm was a way to diminish the intensity of the way they perceived the outer world's madness. For them, it was a coping mechanism but also a combination of most of the other reasons listed above.

The teen I worked with was also working with a therapist, who specialized in managing patients who self-harm. I provided tools to build self-esteem, notice triggers, identify and manage emotions, and adapt other coping mechanisms for self-care. Our work in tandem helped this teen feel more confident, and they have vowed to no longer cut themselves.

One of the tools I used with this teen was to bring constant awareness through self-inquiry to the connection between the behavior, the thought, and their feelings. They set a timer once every two hours on their phone and committed to writing out their answers to these three questions in their journal, each and every day:

- What am I feeling?
- What am I thinking?
- What am I doing?

With these answers, they began to develop a more holistic understanding of how their desire to self-harm was sparked from the emotion, which was then translated into thought, followed by an impulse to carry out the self-harm behavior. However, had the parent not noticed the red flag of self-harming initially and sought help, the teen would not have wanted to do the work to stop participating in this behavior.

Drinking & Drugs

If you are a zero-tolerance parent when it comes to drinking or drugs, this can become a very contentious topic, which means this section just might trigger you. So, take a deep breath before continuing to read on.

As you know, due to hyper-rational thinking and limited impulse control, teenagers often seek thrilling new experiences and are susceptible to the pressures of their peers. If your adolescent is currently drinking or using drugs, your willingness to be open to understanding why they made these choices is of vital importance. If you are shut off to the subject entirely, maintaining a zero-tolerance stance, your teen may feel there is no point in coming clean or engaging in any dialogue with you because they know they will be judged, scorned, or worse – punished.

In his book *Brainstorm: The Power and Purpose of the Teenage Brain*, Dr. Daniel Siegel lays out the four fundamental drives that can motivate increased drug or alcohol use during the adolescent period. These are: experimentation, social connection, self-medication, and addiction. Let's take a look at each of these a little deeper and identify where the red flags are.

- **Experimentation:** One of the main reasons adolescents experiment with drinking or drugs, regardless of their family's stance on the matter, is experimentation: seeking novelty, excitement, or adventure. According to a survey of high school juniors and seniors, 35% have tried alcohol or marijuana, and at least 40% had admitted to being drunk or high over the past year. If you choose to deny the prevalence of drugs or alcohol in normal teen life, this is equivalent to burying your head in the sand and wishing it wasn't so.

- **Peer Pressure:** Another study has revealed that social connection is one of the biggest influences prompting teens to use drugs or alcohol. In essence, teens want to be part of the social fabric of shared experiences in certain circles and settings. At events, such as parties and concerts, drinking alcohol or smoking marijuana may be an expected behavior. Additionally, teens express drugs or alcohol help lower social anxiety and personal defenses that help them feel more at ease in social settings, acting as a social lubricant.

- **Using to Numb:** Drug and alcohol use can transform into an act of self-medicating to avoid emotional distress. Adolescents who suffer from depression, anxiety, or any other countless disorders may find drugs or alcohol as an easier path to escape rather than dealing with their challenges. A habit of avoidance could lead to using drugs and alcohol as a further means of avoidance.

- **Addiction:** This usually starts with one of the other reasons above and progresses. In order for a person to feel higher, more buzzed, or whatever the desired effect is, an increased amount of drugs or alcohol may be needed. Perhaps the use of a particular drug or alcohol no longer delivers the same results, so the adolescent may move on to using them more frequently, using them in greater quantities, or gravitate towards more dangerous substances. The brain can become dependent on the chemical release and may start to crave this reaction into a state of dependence.

Have a conversation with your teen, explore these four drives to use drugs or alcohol, and share your desire to create a safe space to talk about it without judgment. If you suspect your teen is using drugs or alcohol as a way to numb or has become addicted, those are red flags you cannot ignore.

Sex

With adolescence arrives the new sensations of puberty, sexual arousal, romantic interests, and gender roles and identities, all of which can be uncomfortable or confusing. The newness of these sensations correlates with the adolescent brain's desire for novelty. Experiencing these new feelings and developing the desire to explore these natural sensations is not, in itself, a red flag, but a natural part of maturing.

Many parents have rigid beliefs about what is appropriate to discuss or consider with their teens and what is not. These beliefs become an obstacle if you cannot talk candidly with your teen about this subject. With your approval or permission or not, teens are having sex more often than you think.

According to one study, more than half of U.S. teens have had sexual intercourse before the age of 18. Another study in the UK reveals teenage pregnancy rates are rising in the 13 - 15 year age group. This study reveals that twenty percent of 13-year-olds surveyed said they had already had either full sexual intercourse or oral sex with a partner. The study shows that adolescents as young as 12 or 13 years old becoming fully sexually active is trending upwards.

Sex among younger teens is a concern and, of course, a red flag. One of the common reasons for choosing to have sex at an early age is increased peer pressure, adventure and excitement, and a deep desire to feel wanted and loved. Many of these young people don't fully understand the ideas surrounding consent, sexual preference, and gender identities, nor do they feel empowered to say "no" without feeling judged. As you can imagine, high-risk behavior, especially among younger adolescents, can lead to unwanted pregnancies, exposure to sexually transmitted diseases, and placing themselves in potentially dangerous situations. Another risk among teens of all ages is not having access to care for the medical consequences of risky sexual behavior.

The teens I've worked with over the last ten years have talked about the predominant culture of hookups. Hookups are casual encounters with multiple partners that have a high focus on physical satisfaction and completely ignore the emotional and mental side of intimacy. Many of the girls I've worked with explain how peer pressure surrounding hookup culture normalizes treating one's body as a vehicle for pleasure for themselves and their partners. Most of the teens I've talked to about this have never once considered the emotional implications of this behavior. Another problem with hookup culture is the inequality of expectations and emotions. I've worked with many teens who've felt rejected, unlovable, unworthy, and ugly because a causal hookup partner no longer wants to have sex with them.

Reds flags surrounding sex, sexual activity, hookups, and intimacy run the gamut and will be as individual as your teen is. As the parent, you have no choice but to take the lead and create connections around these topics. Please have conversations, define safe spaces, have an open mind, and connect with your adolescent deep and often. Do not be afraid to intervene when you suspect there may be a red flag waving for you to see.

What to Do if You Notice These Red Flags

Each of the red flags in this chapter has its own appropriate response, but in general, your job is to keep communication constant, open, and honest. Red flags may be a warning signal to look at a particular circumstance as a literal life or death situation. Your teen needs to know you are their beacon and they can come to you about everything. You need to make a commitment to yourself to broach uncomfortable topics openly and often with your adolescent. Share your own experiences and fears when you were their age and let them know what red flags you are concerned about. Let your teen know they are not alone and their experiences are not unique.

Here are some quick reminders of how to respond when you notice a red flag:

- **Be rational.** First and foremost, manage your own emotional state. Never approach your teen when you are dysregulated. Talk to your teen rationally, with kindness and compassion, and don't go on the attack.

- **Listen.** Use empathy and listen without judgment. Make it a priority to understand their point of view. Ask them to share their emotions, fears, and beliefs about the situation. Try to get a clearer image of what their world looks like from their vantage point.

- **Educate yourself.** Understand all the topics explored in this chapter, mental health disorders and challenges, are 100% treatable. Learn about the specific topic in detail and educate yourself about treatment, options, approaches, and responses.

- **Enlist support from other adults.** If a teen doesn't open up to you, enlist the help of other adults in their life, such as family friends, coaches, and other trusted relatives. Difficult situations may have unfamiliar roads to navigate, and many teens may feel more comfortable opening up to someone who is not their parent.

- **Guarantee reprieve.** Make sure your teen knows they will *not* be punished. You shouldn't be punishing anyway if you are practicing partnership parenting. Encourage honesty and open dialogue without the fear of judgment. Assure your teen that you are not seeking intimate details. Communicate that you are trying to understand the feelings behind their actions or choices and that your only intention is to support or help them in the best way possible.

- **Find a professional.** If the situation doesn't improve, I recommend finding a therapist, practitioner, or treatment plan. Parents should do this immediately if their teen appears to be at risk of harming themselves or others.

Chapter 8: Why Tools?

That uneasy feeling washed over me again, starting from the back of my neck, rising up to the top of my head, then pouring down as heat into my forehead and cheeks. The driver dropped us off at the corner, and from the moment I stepped off the bus and headed toward my house, the sensations intensified. I had an uncanny knack of knowing when there would be trouble at home and when it felt neutral. This day, I felt those warning signs in my body as the feeling of dread swelled within me with each step I took.

I was thirteen, and life at home was mostly unbearable. Thick tension, high stress, and feelings of being judged would propel me into a constant state of flight, flight, or freeze. But I was grateful I had these skills. This was how I survived.

To an outsider, the patterns in our home must have been predictable. The tensions between my mother and myself would build over time, then there was a massive blowup. Our blowups weren't necessarily over a "thing" that happened or something I did wrong, but part of our natural cycle. It felt more like a pressure cooker about ready to blow, and the "thing" would be found to justify the blowup. Each engagement felt like a struggle over power and control, and I could always feel them coming on. Because I would not stand down, my strong will always enraged my mother further.

This particular day, as I approached my house, my intuition told me this was going to be one of those days. When I entered the house, my mother was in my room waiting for me. She had pulled into the center of my bedroom the large metal trash can, which normally lived on the side of the house.

I had a collection of bottles displayed by size, shape, and color on the bookshelf above my desk. I had saved the bottles from the wine my parents drank and found other colored bottles from around the neighborhood. I had blue, green, brown, and clear bottles. I had spent hours soaking the bottles and removing the labels and glue from each of them.

My mother was waiting for me. I noticed she had one of my bottles in her hand. She was hostile and started yelling, but I can't recall what she was saying. I remember the rage in her eyes as she smashed the first bottle with immense force inside the metal bin. The loud crash reverberated in my bedroom, and I jumped back.

Then, with calculating purpose, my mother pulled each bottle off the shelf, one by one, and violently smashed them into the bin. I remember screaming for her to stop, but the crashing and smashing sounds within the metal can were deafening...

I replayed this incident over and over in my mind numerous times over the last forty years. The effects of that incident left a deep scar on me. However, I learned through tools to use this as one of my baseline events to track my own healing.

When I was nineteen years old, I participated in one of those "human potential" seminars, which were immensely popular in the sixties, seventies, and eighties. The Human Potential Movement arose out of the counterculture of the sixties and formed around the concept that each one of us has extraordinary potential inside of us that can be tapped into. We just need to tap into it!

I attended a weekend gathering, offered through the company Lifespring. Although I only attended Level 1 and never went through their full program, this was my first exposure to self-advocacy, self-healing, and the use of a variety of tools to do so. Throughout the weekend, I was exposed to many systems and tools for healing. One of the tools I was introduced to was called the Wheel of Life, which I'll share in the next chapter.

I've used tools in my own healing and within my practice with teens for many, many years. Tools provide a methodical, external method to process and track our internal worlds. Tools encourage us to go deeper through self-inquiry and observation and help us to know ourselves better from the inside out. Tools also present a neutral, judgment-free experience, meaning the tools don't criticize us. They are simply a platform for us to examine what's there. Good tools provide an equally objective and subjective guide for reflection.

Through tools, I was able to uncover how the incident I shared above affected me and empowered me to observe patterns of beliefs to track my own healing.

For example, I learned to track occurrences of emotions and uncover the anchored beliefs using tools. The emotions I felt, as a result of the bottle smashing incident, were fear, violation, betrayal, confusion, sadness, grief, vulnerability, and despair.

From those feelings, the beliefs I developed, or the beliefs that became reinforced, were: *People will violate and betray me, I am unlovable, I cannot trust people to be fair,* and *I am not worthy of kindness.* Now, I have an easier time identifying triggers that activate those old patterns of beliefs when I feel these emotions. That kind of awareness helps me heal each and every day.

By having tools available to use, you can jump-start healing processes in yourself and your adolescent, which can support reprogramming old habits or beliefs that no longer serve us. Furthermore, once you find a tool that works for you, it's yours for life. As a parent, using tools together with your teen places you into the role of partnership on their mental health journey as opposed to directing it.

Facilitation

In Chapter 2, we introduced the differences between teaching and facilitation, explored the value of modeling, and talked about using the tool of connection over coercion. If you haven't figured it out by now, facilitation is actually the art and act of partnering.

Your role as a facilitator will require you to commit to being an empathetic listener by practicing the ability to reflect on what you have heard from your teen and will require, from you, the patience of a saint.

Facilitating the tools in this book with your adolescent will require a great deal of self-awareness. Stepping into the role of a facilitator is not easy, especially since we, as parents, are emotionally entangled with our child's well-being. Maintaining objectivity will require an extra layer of self-control on our behalf. One of the themes throughout his book has been becoming responsible and hyper-aware when your own beliefs or fears creep into your engagement with your teen. These beliefs can be translated into expectations or agendas, which can color your ability to facilitate. Your own emotional intelligence will be tested, as will your ability to identify, manage, and regulate your own triggers or defensiveness. Once you comfortably feel you have mastered these skills, you are ready to (deep breath) facilitate.

As the facilitator, you must be keenly sensitive not to put your teen in a position to defend themselves. When your teen shares thoughts, feelings, and experiences that are uncomfortable for you, do whatever you can to put your teen at ease. If they feel judged, they will certainly shut down. Your job is to build trust and a strong connection. Sometimes we have the tendency to reply to self-deprecating thoughts with "That's not true, honey. You are _____ (smart, likable, pretty, etc.)." As much as we believe whatever they just said is not actually true, we must never say those words. This invalidates their thoughts. Instead, we must find the language to help them unpack those thoughts in order for them to make their own self-discoveries. Not seeing, hearing, or understanding their thoughts will close the connection right then and there. Please, recognize this is hard work.

Another directive the facilitator must follow is not offering opinions or feedback. That's super difficult for many of us, but remember, you are not there to solve their problems. You are there to facilitate your teen's self-exploration. The only time it is acceptable to offer up advice is when your teen specifically asks for it. Even then, you must be prepared and willing to accept if your teen chooses not to take the advice you offered.

The last factor you must consider is not all teens want to be facilitated by their parents. It's just a fact. Adolescence is a time of individualization, and the connection our children once had with us could now be focused on other people: other significant adults in their lives, coaches, or mentors who they feel safe opening up with. We'll explore more about the benefits of mentoring in the last chapter. If your adolescent does not want to be facilitated by you, you must not take it personally. Forcing a connection when they are resisting can create a fracture in your connection. My advice in this situation is to keep finding ways to connect with your teen through vulnerability by sharing your own self-discoveries and modeling patience, compassion, and kindness. They will notice it.

Milestones

Milestones are reference points to note where you are in the life cycle of whatever it is you are measuring. Milestones help us keep track of the important stages of progress. Milestones can be set up to help you evaluate incremental progress while having clearly defined checkpoints to ensure you're headed in the right direction.

Standardized milestones are used in project development, mental and physical health plans, and within many branches of scientific research. You can even find lists of standard milestones to define states of human growth and development. We can apply the same idea to our own self-directed healing path and the healing path of our adolescents.

In order to know if we are progressing, we need to have a clear idea of the point we are starting from. The self-assessment form found in the beginning of Chapter 9 will help you track your progress and develop your own milestones. One recommendation for using the tools in the next chapter is to create your own milestones to monitor how both you and your teen are doing. If you decide to practice the tools in this book on yourself before facilitating these tools with your teen, tracking your progress will provide inspiration for both of you. Sharing these outcomes with your teen is not only a way to inspire them, but it can provide an avenue to connect deeper. It's a win-win, right?

As you know, adolescence is a time of changes: changes in the way they think, feel, and interact with others, and changes in how their bodies are transforming. Teens are busy developing unique personalities, opinions, and interests to create a clearer sense of who they are. They are also preparing for greater independence and responsibility.

Let's look at common developmental milestones in adolescents and line them up with the mental health goals you may suggest for your teens. Although all the tools in the next chapter can be used with adolescents of all ages, the developmental milestones may make some of the tools more challenging depending on where they are in their own growth milestones.

Emotional, Social, & Cognitive Milestones During Adolescence

Developmental Milestone	Tool	Desired Milestone
Concrete, black-and-white thinking (early adolescence)	Self-assessment	Developing skills to objectively know one's self
Self-conscious (early adolescence)	Wheel of Life	Identifying areas in one's life that need focus
Abstract thinking (late adolescence)	Self-inquiry	Adapting self-inquiry as a daily practice
Hyperrational thinking	Beliefs	Pausing before acting

Greater intensity of feelings	Triggers	Managing triggers
Struggling with personal identity	Masks	Showing self more authentically
Engage in risk-taking activities that provide emotional intensity	Reframing	Being accountable & making responsible choices
Think abstractly and consider the big picture (middle adolescence)	Shadow Work	Developing a holistic sense of self
Self-doubt, self-esteem, and self-confidence	Fear	Choosing responses to fear versus being stuck in "reaction mode"
Be better able to give reasons for their own choices, including what is right or wrong	Core Values	Living from a place of values
Thinks about different possibilities and begins to develop their own identity	Worldviews	Developing compassion

Planning for future	Passion & Purpose	Choices based on passion & purpose
Self-image, self-identity (negative or positive) is largely formed based on experience and perception of one's "place"	People Pleasing	Creating boundaries, developing a voice
Show more independence from parents	Goals & Accountability	Executing and meeting goals
Conflicts & disagreements	Conflict Resolution	Resolving conflicts intentionally
Learn more defined habits	Self-Care	Daily self-care practices
Hyperrationality	Pause	Practicing pausing
Experimentation (drugs, alcohol, sex, etc.)	Connection through trust	Accountability and honesty

One of the tools I've used in my Transformative Mentoring for Teens courses is tasking teens with a challenge to decorate a shoebox that demonstrates their taste, likes, values, and their artistic skills. This decorated shoebox becomes a gift they are preparing for themselves and a way for them to track their own milestones.

At the end of my course, I ask the teens to place all the tools, worksheets, reflections, and journal entries they've completed over the past few months into the box. The final challenge is asking the teens to write a letter to their future self and add it to the box, which will be opened one year from the date of our last meeting.

This process creates a literal milestone, marking who they are now and recording the expectation they have for who they wish to become in one year. Through this act, teens are intentionally creating a symbolic milestone. Recognizing our own mental health awareness and tracking how our lives improve as a result automatically becomes another important milestone.

Highly-Engaged States

When we are highly engaged (alert and learning), natural chemical reactions are taking place in the brain. Learning a little about these processes can assist us in creating optimal environments for learning, exploring, and healing. In Chapter 6, we explored the effects of dopamine on the adolescent brain. In this section, we're going to take a closer look at some of the other contributing hormones that affect brain chemistry in relation to creating highly-engaged states.

Researchers believe the brain chemicals that influence students in a traditional classroom setting are serotonin, dopamine, cortisol, and norepinephrine. According to Eric Jensen, a brain-based education expert, stimulating those four neurotransmitters can lead to the brain being fully engaged, therefore creating an optimal environment for learning. We are going to borrow from this theory in order to assist parents everywhere to create the best environments to help their adolescents learn and explore their inner worlds.

Serotonin: Setting the Mood

The neurotransmitter serotonin is responsible for mood regulation. Researchers believe that by creating positive learning rituals involving comfort, familiarity, and aesthetically-pleasing surroundings can boost serotonin levels.

In the acclaimed book, *The Highly Engaged Classroom*, the authors report students in classrooms are better primed to learn if their surroundings are warm and welcoming. You can translate this into your own serotonin-boosting response by selecting a comfortable neutral space as your dedicated zone for your inner journey together. Create your unique ritual. Pour a cup of warm tea and find a cozy spot in your garden, an overstuffed couch at your local cafe, or a sunny breakfast nook. Approach this space with positivity and enthusiasm, which will set the mood and enhance emotional bonds by increasing serotonin levels.

Cortisol: Stress Responses

If you or your teen are in a state of high stress, this is not an optimal time to focus on using tools. Do whatever you can to regulate your nervous systems and reschedule your time together.

Cortisol is the hormone associated with stress regulation. Though it's challenging to measure cortisol levels and correlate those amounts with specific outcomes, there are a few ways researchers have determined how cortisol affects the brain. Cortisol is known as the messenger hormone, whose job it is to transmit a set of instructions from one part of the body to the next. The messages delivered are often critical and designed to set off a chain of biochemical events, depending on the "content" of the message.

Chronic stress and high levels of cortisol can influence cognition. High levels of stress can affect the way you think, contribute to poor memory, make simple tasks more difficult, and negatively harm the body.

However, researchers acknowledge that low levels of stress (and cortisol) have positive effects on learning. Naturally, as the brain encounters novel or challenging experiences, it is acquiring new information, which is generating low levels of stress in the brain. Stress itself is not inherently bad; stress is intrinsic to our ability to learn and grow. In order to create highly-engaged states to learn, we must have low levels of cortisol, but it's vital we keep this balanced.

Dopamine: Rewards and Pleasures

The tools in this book are designed to generate new insights about ourselves, thus stimulating the rewards centers of our teens' brains through each new discovery. Uncovering new insights is rewarding and feels good. When we experience rewards, the brain can be flooded with dopamine, giving us a feeling of satisfaction and pleasure. As dopamine levels increase in the brain, the new information we are learning becomes anchored in our memory through our emotions.

Another discovery we can borrow from highly-engaged classrooms is the strategy of including unpredictable moments to help keep the excitement growing and the pleasure center activated. One strategy is adding music, which helps to create a more imaginative environment. These pleasurable moments allow the brain to be more receptive to information because dopamine levels have risen.

Norepinephrine: Moving and Learning

Norepinephrine affects many areas of the brain, such as the amygdala, which can influence where we direct our attention. When norepinephrine is released, we are less distracted and focus occurs. The part of the brain that processes movement is also the same part that processes learning. Therefore, not sitting too long and getting up to physically moving every ten minutes or so can make all the difference in releasing norepinephrine and other transmitters, thus helping adolescents retain learning and increasing focus and engagement.

Remember this, when your adolescent is in a highly-engaged state, both future goals and self-inquiry goals have a totally different feeling and focus. The exercise of knowing and understanding what that feels like creates a familiar feeling. The chemical releases can activate urgency and focus and help our teens to process more effectively.

Best Practices Using Tools

Perfect mental health has always been, and will likely always be, out of one's reach because it doesn't exist. The goal of this book is not to fix a person, but rather to provide a greater understanding of how tools can assist each one of us living our best lives. There will always be struggles. There will always be challenges. Such is the nature of life. There will never be a point where you will say, "I'm done. I've achieved perfect mental health."

For those of us who experienced traumas, those things will always be with us. For those of us who developed untrue limiting beliefs about ourselves, we will never eradicate them from our memories. For those of us who have deep haunting shadows, we will never erase them. Tools are designed to help us live in partnership with ourselves unconditionally. Tools can help us to understand ourselves better and choose how we respond to the programming we've endured. Tools can improve the quality of our lives and help us manage mental illness, stressors, and fears. But we are the "us" we are, and tools will not help us escape that. However, they will help us to accept that and assist us in choosing who we want to become.

Before you jump into the tools, please consider some of these best practices. Not each suggestion will be a match for you or your teen, so please feel free to throw out anything that is not in alignment with your unique way of being in this world.

1. **Create routines.** For some people, creating routines can stimulate improvement in their state of mental health. Setting alarms, making a calendar, and developing routines that vary hourly, daily, weekly, and monthly can help us stay calm and focused.

2. **Set goals.** Creating goals, defining milestones, and creating an overall schedule can help us stimulate dopamine releases, which will help to keep us focused and motivated. Start small with daily goals such as journaling, taking a class, or using one of the tools in this book. Then, you can build up into larger goals like learning a new skill. Goal setting is super important for finding meaning, especially

in those who suffer from depression or anxiety. Having something to look forward to, something to strive towards, to work towards, makes a world of difference in our overall mental health.

3. **Manage your physical health.** Eating healthy, exercising, good hygiene, and getting sufficient sleep all to contribute to your overall mental wellness. Go for daily walks and get into a routine for general self-care.

4. **Be kind to yourself.** This is one we all slip up on. Use tools when we notice we are in a pattern of negative thinking, record and manage our triggers, and most of all, use tools to control our self-sabotaging behavior and thoughts.

5. **Prioritize yourself.** Take care of your needs before focusing on someone else's. Make sure you are not people-pleasing and get into a practice of prioritizing yourself first. Perform self-checks and ask yourself questions such as, "Do I really want to do this?" "Am I saying yes out of obligation?" or "Is this decision best for **me**?"

6. **Surround yourself with positive people.** Choose to surround yourself with people who are positive influences and can help outweigh the negative influences in your life. Learning to advocate for yourself is essential. Communicate effectively and create boundaries with people who are not positive in your life by articulating what you will and will not tolerate.

7. **Try new things.** Get into the habit of stepping outside of your comfort zone, learning to feel comfortable with the discomfort, and trying new things. Teens' brains are wired for novelty so learning to manage the fear and negative self-talk is essential.

8. **Celebrate the little wins.** Just as achieving goals, when we celebrate the little wins, we are instigating dopamine releases in the brain. As we know, dopamine releases feel good. Allowing ourselves to celebrate even the smallest of wins, we will stay motivated and on track.

9. **Remove yourself from unhealthy situations.** As we are learning to advocate for ourselves, removing ourselves from situations that are unhealthy, dangerous, and stressful will create a practice of self-advocacy. However, we must be able to differentiate discomfort from stress, and that requires self-inquiry.

10. **Develop positive coping skills.** Define your own library of coping skills, like relaxing your stomach when you're panicking, deep breathing exercises, meditation, yoga, distraction tolerance, or mindfulness. Discover what works best for you and know what your go-to practices are for coping and regulating your nervous system.

11. **Eliminate stress.** Do you feel overtasked or overwhelmed? Take a step back and reevaluate what exactly you need in your life and what is unnecessary. Don't take on things that could eliminate "you" time, and don't unnecessarily stress yourself out. Taking on too much at once can add to undo stress.

12. **Welcome change.** Do not fear change. Change is a part of life, and building skills to deal with change will help you to build resiliency. Create an even balance between change and routine to help you build skills to better manage chaos and peace equally.

13. **Take care of yourself.** Love yourself. Embrace yourself. Use tools. Use tools often. Do not look at yourself as if something is wrong; instead, look at yourself as being uniquely you. You may never have perfect mental health, but you can be happy.

Chapter 9: Tools

"My daughter was so blown away by the tools Lainie uses she said she felt like she was skydiving in her head."
~ Taryn Helper, Parent

I'm so excited to finally get to this chapter, aren't you? We have spoken about so many different facets of adolescent development, the teen brain, your role in partnering, and so much more! This chapter is where all that information comes together, and we start to apply everything we've learned through action.

I've recommended that parents should always try the tools in this book first before facilitating them with their teens. Once you are fully aware of how they function and the emotions they uncover, you will be in a better place to facilitate with compassion, candor, and vulnerability. In order for any tool to work, your teen must fully opt-in and consent to do this work; otherwise, the tools will not be effective.

Another approach you could try, whether you go through the exercises alone first or not, would be to do this work as a family. This will once again depend on the willingness of your teen and whether having both parents and possibly siblings present for the exercises would make them more or less comfortable. Give your teen the option of what would work best for them, then respect and honor that decision by following through without letting your own emotions get in the way.

One of the last best pieces of advice I can give to you before diving into the tools is to urge you to create a practice of journaling. Journal daily, and journal often. Journal after each of the tools, journal reflections, new discoveries, and insights. Get it out and onto paper.

Invite your teen to journal as well and encourage them to keep it private, letting them know this is for their eyes and their eyes only. And of course, you should never breach that boundary. Reflecting through writing helps us process, and the act of using our hands to write our thoughts, versus typing on our phones or computers, helps us to slow down our thoughts and attach a physical action to our processing.

Remember, there are never wrong answers when you're working with these tools. Simply recording how you think, feel, and process in this present moment of NOW. These tools are timeless. Do the same exercise three months from now, six months later, or even a year from now. You will see how your state of understanding and awareness will change.

You must also commit to being in a state of non-judgment and fully accept whatever comes up for you and your teen. Recognize your own journey to this point and recognize the journey your teen has taken to get here. Establish the boundaries of a safe space and invite the possibility of change, growth, and healing as your highest intention.

In my practice, I use numerous tools to support the mental health of adolescents (and sometimes parents). I've selected the most powerful ones to get you started. Ready? Let's jump right in!

Self-Assessment

Knowing where you are starting from helps you to know where you want to go. Please use the answers in this self-assessment exercise to start your own three-month set of goals.

You are invited to answer the questions below as honestly and authentically as possible. This form is a tool for you as you begin to embark on your journey inward and truly know yourself. By making a commitment to fill out this questionnaire with honesty, you are setting the stage for your own transformation. You are always in the driver's seat.

Let's do this!

Name: Date:	
What 3 outcomes would you most like to achieve over the next 3-6 months?	1. 2. 3.

List 3 issues, concerns, worries, or challenges within yourself that you wish to address, understand, change, or transform over the next 3 months?

1.	
2.	
3.	

Why do you desire to take action now on these issues that are of concern or interest to you?

What actions have you taken in the past (whether on your own initiative or with support) to address these issues and with what success?

What are the qualities, strengths, and values that you have, which you think will be most helpful towards achieving the outcomes you have set out in the first question, above?

Qualities:	
Strengths:	
Values:	

What are your 3 biggest worries as to what might stop you from achieving the outcomes you are looking for?

Worry 1:	
Worry 2:	
Worry 3:	

Given your answers to the questions above, list a small number of actions (imagined or not) that you can now take to begin to move towards the outcomes that you would like to achieve or deal with your concerns, worries, or challenges:

1.	
2.	
3.	
4.	

5.

What are the most important things in your life?

What would you do with your life if you were guaranteed success?

What needs of yours would you be meeting by doing what you described above (in the "if you were guaranteed success" question)?

What are the biggest obstacles in your way preventing you from doing what you want to do (if you were guaranteed success)?

Self-Inquiry

We've spoken about self-inquiry at length throughout this book. In Chapter 4, I introduced you to Byron Katie's *The Work*, which is a wonderful way to get familiar with and practice a self-inquiry process.

Before we dig into the next tool, I want to explain why self-inquiry is important and why you must become familiar with the process of checking inward before responding in any situation. Many of us never actually respond because we are programmed to "react." Our reactions are learned auto-responses, which come from our early childhood, traumas, and a lifetime of experiences. Reacting from the beliefs formed in the mind of a three-year-old girl may not be an appropriate reaction in our adult situations. Become fluent in self-inquiry. Pausing when we experience dysregulating thoughts, feelings, and beliefs and inquiring about what is happening in our internal worlds can help us break the habit of being in an auto-response mode.

Self-inquiry can bridge the conscious-thinking mind with the unconscious and the subconscious mind. We have access to the unconscious part of the brain, but it takes practice to build the pathways. Self-inquiry is one of the best tools to improve that connection.

The first step of self-inquiry is noticing when we have a reaction to a situation. Is this reaction identifiable? Can we name our emotions? Can we notice the physical reaction? Can we determine *where* in our body we are feeling our reaction? Does this feeling we've just identified have a belief below it or attached to it? Are there layers of emotions stacked onto our beliefs? It's likely so.

Here are the simple steps to practice self-inquiry:

> What is the thought? (Name it.)
> What is the feeling? (Use the emotions wheel in Chapter 2.)
> Where is the feeling residing in your body? (Name the body part and the physical sensation.)

What meaning does this have? (Name the new thought.)
Repeat as many times as you can. (GO DEEP)
Write down your process, keep a journal, date it, review it, get familiar, and learn your patterns.

Here is an example a parent might experience after their teen walks in from the day, ignores them, then proceeds to walk past them without a word:

> You may notice the thought, "My teen always treats me like I don't matter," Then the feelings this brings up are rejection, anger, and frustration. Then, you may notice your heart feels heavy and your stomach tightens. After, you identify the emotion of deep disappointment, attached to numbing and sadness. The next belief you notice attached to that combination of feelings is, "I feel I am a failure as a parent."
>
> Then, start the process over again. Define where that feeling is sitting in your body and repeat. In the end, you may discover you have a deep-seated belief that maybe you learned early on you were unlovable or not worthy of being loved. Whatever it is, don't be afraid of uncovering what's there.

Once you go down three to five layers and start to uncover the hidden items causing some issues, you will have awareness of the subconscious thoughts auto-prompting you to react. You'll start to notice your thoughts and patterns and how they affect your behavior in certain situations. This can then help you to consciously choose an appropriate response instead. It's really empowering, I promise!

Learning to pause is really the first step in your own empowerment, which is why a family that pauses together grows together. It's important to note the goal is not to rid the mind of our programming but to make peace with it, recognize it's there, and create the skills through self-inquiry to program new alternate options (writing new neural pathways).

The key is to use the first trigger, thought, or emotion as a tool to guide you to recognize what is below that. As we dig down through those layers of beliefs and traumas, it will not be easy, and the results won't be linear.

Here is an example of what we might uncover as we drill down into the layers, but it can start from anyplace:

- Trigger
- Core belief
- Emotion
- Core belief
- Trigger

In my programs, I use worksheets to help us get comfortable diving deeper and getting comfortable with self-inquiry. The process can be done on our own, of course, but facilitated self-inquiry or having the support of someone else to help us unpack what we wrote is always more powerful. Give this simple self-inquiry tool a try:

What 3 issues are showing up NOW in my life that have me frustrated, hurting, or upset that I want to change?	
Issue, challenge, or frustration #1:	
Issue, challenge, or frustration #2:	

Issue, challenge, or frustration #3:	

What link(s) do I find between these three challenges or frustrations?

What do the link(s) or pattern(s) say to me about who I am?

How does this pattern keep showing up in my life?

What have I tried to do to overcome this pattern?

Who would I be without these challenges, frustrations, and patterns?

Describe my desired outcome and how I can imagine it changing my life:

Why do I want to change these patterns, frustrations, and challenges?

How do these patterns stop me from…	
…accomplishing my dreams and goals?	
…being more loving and available to the people in my life?	
…being healthy and relaxed?	
…being able to be an active contributor in my own life?	
…feeling confident and in control of my life?	

What matters to me most?

What emotions do I feel when the pattern is playing out in my life?

What have I noticed about myself by examining my patterns, challenges, and frustrations?

Wheel of Life

Another really great tool to use to evaluate where you currently are on your life's journey is called the Wheel of Life. This powerful tool helps you visually assess your life, create milestones, and understand which areas in your life to prioritize. The original concept is attributed to the late Paul J. Meyer, who founded the Success Motivation Institute in 1960. I was first introduced to this tool when I was 19 and always found it a wonderful way to gauge where I was in order to know where I wanted to go. This tool is very popular among life coaches and transformational coaches.

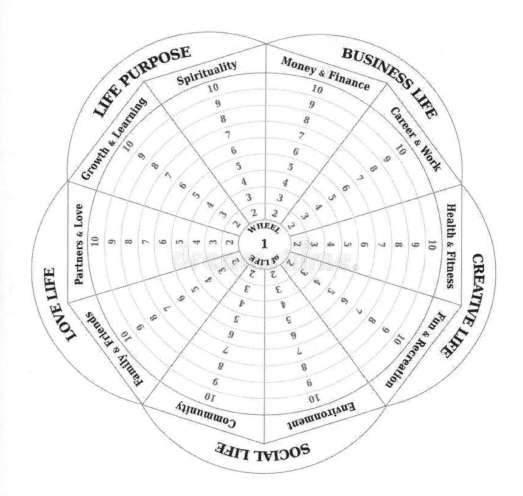

How to Use the Wheel of Life

The Wheel of Life can be customized to fit your own needs, lifestyle, or current challenges.

1. **Determine your categories.** Identify the areas in your life where you devote most of your time. Each person is going to be different, but there are some general areas to choose from. These prompts will help

you define the categories most important. In the case of working with your adolescent, be flexible and customize according to their lead:

- List out the most important areas of your life. This may include education, job or career, family, friends, community & social contributions, finances, health, and creative projects.
- Choose the most important roles in your life. Some of the roles you might identify could be a friend, daughter/son/child, community leader, volunteer, artist/musician, athlete, student, team member, boyfriend/girlfriend/partner, etc.
- Identify the overlap from your previous list. This will help you to reflect on all the areas of your life that you consider a priority, such as a volunteer role in your community that allows you to use your creative talents.

2. **Create a wheel using the categories you chose.** Once you have decided on your categories, you can create a diagram design and label each space between the spokes of your wheel of life. You can even artistically design your own version or use a simple one like the one above.

3. **Evaluate each area.** The concept behind the Wheel of Life is that you can find fulfillment and happiness if you can find the right balance among your categories. You'll want to use your wheel of life to visually determine how much time is being devoted to each of the important areas of your life. Go through each category and rank how much attention you're currently devoting on a scale of 0 to 10, with 0 being the lowest and 10 being the highest. Once you determine a category's score, write it down and mark it in the corresponding space. Consider what your ideal attention level is for each category, then plot those scores on your wheel of life in a different color.

4. **Connect the dots.** After you have gone through each category and marked your score on your wheel of life, connect each mark around the circle. Is it even or is it unbalanced? By connecting the dots, you

can see just how each area compares and decide whether your wheel appears to be balanced for you.

5. **Compare the results to your ideal levels.** It's true, different areas of your life will require different amounts of attention. In other words, achieving a balanced life doesn't have to mean you need to give an equal amount of time or focus to each category.

6. **Make a plan to improve specific areas in your life.** Notice any gaps that exist between your current life and ideal life balance. It's possible, there could be areas where you just don't have the time to devote your desired amount of attention. That's ok. In fact, that's life!

Using this visual tool, you can identify the gaps. The Wheel of Life provides a personalized visual map of how to help you make decisions based on your priorities by assisting you to consciously decide which areas in your life you are choosing to give more attention to.

Triggers

In Chapter 4, we explored triggers and accountability, but this tool will help us to go a little deeper. Triggers are reactions, which are generally emotional in nature. They tap into our beliefs and can be activated at any given moment, especially if something is pushing up against our core beliefs. The trigger can generate an emotional reaction in our bodies. Much of the programming in this regard comes from an autopilot process similar to fight, flight, or freeze.

The first part is recognizing the trigger that set us off, especially if we are triggered often. We can do this by tracking the thoughts, actions, and behaviors that led to this response. Oftentimes, if we don't get a better handle on what's going on, this can lead to damaging behavior on our part. When we are aware of what is happening, we can then choose a response instead of letting our body just react.

The second part is using the tools in this chapter to help our teens recognize the first step of their trigger process so over time, they can do the work of self-inquiry by uncovering what the belief below the emotion is.

You can use this next tool in conjunction with the trigger log I provided back in Chapter 4. After you and your teen have become comfortable tracking your triggers, this next tool will help you to go deeper and unpack their effects. You can recreate this tool below and have several copies ready to use as triggers occur. It's always most effective using this tool as near to the event as possible.

Date of trigger:	
Time of occurrence:	
Describe what happened in three sentences or less:	
How did I react in the moment?	

Three emotions I immediately felt as I was triggered were:	1. 2. 3.
Three secondary emotions I am feeling now, as I am processing the event are:	1. 2. 3.
In less than three sentences, describe: I am noticing I am feeling different now about…	
The belief this incident challenged is:	

Masks

This is one of my favorite tools, and this is the first tool we use together in my group. The feedback I get after using this tool is always insightful and filled with aha moments.

Masks, every person out there uses them to one degree or another. We put on different masks for different occasions. Just as archetypes, we use masks for two reasons: to hide a part of ourselves or to become something else we are not, borrowing some attribute from an alternate identity. Either way, people commonly mask themselves without knowing it.

Start off with this simple template on the next page. Ask yourself or your teen, "What mask are you wearing right now?" Then, in the oval shape, draw the simple attributes that represent the mask. Is it smiling or is it unhappy? Is it dramatic, based on a character, or is it nondescript? Is revealing emotions, filled with color, or is it closed off? Is it something you normally are not or is your normal "go-to" in this situation mask? Even if you don't identify as artistic, allow yourself to artistically explore the mask you are wearing right at this moment.

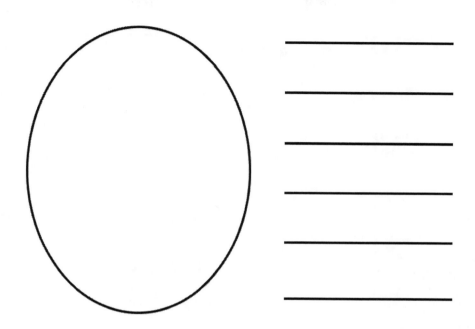

With the lines beside the mask, write a simple bulleted list of the qualities and attributes of that mask. Simple is fine, but make sure you write what you see.

After you've explored the mask you are wearing now, ask this question, "What is this mask hiding?" This tool requires reflection, self-inquiry, and of course, journaling.

What purpose do masks serve? Think about this question and fill out the following tool based on your own experiences.

Occasions I Wear Masks	Name of Mask	Qualities of the Mask	Part of True Self I Am Hiding
school	student mask	complicit, rule follower	rebellious
with friends	bff mask	Likable, supportive, people-pleasing	jealous, afraid of not being accepted

Your responses to this tool can be repeated, reviewed often, and journaled about. The more we know about ourselves, the more we can make choices about how we wish to experience certain situations and life in general. It becomes a milestone when we enter a familiar situation and choose not to wear that mask anymore.

Reframing

This is a super simple tool and also super effective. One of the young adults I've worked with for over a year has shared with me that this is the single most applied tool that she practices over and over, and it has changed her life. Her conscious choice to reframe while she is in the middle of a challenge has always had a calming effect on her, her nervous system, and her overall state of well-being. I can't recommend this practice enough.

So much of our happiness depends on how we choose to look at the world.

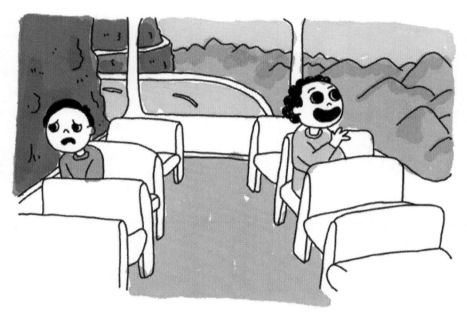

In order to introduce this tool, you are invited to answer three questions, one from the past, one from the present, and one for the future. Please write down your answers to the following questions in your journal or in the notes section at the back of this book:

1. The Past: Write down the worst thing that has happened to you in the last six months or the biggest mistake you've made.

2. The Present: Write down the thing or situation that currently frustrates you or that you perceive as being impossible or majorly difficult.
3. The Future: Finally, write down something you have coming up in the future that hasn't yet taken place, which is a major choice or decision you are faced with.

The Past: The best way to reframe something in your past is to read the statement you wrote down, then ask yourself, "How is this REALLY the best thing that has ever happened to me?" Really think about this question and write down five solid reasons why this thing that happened to you in the past was really a tremendous gift or opportunity. Search your mind, find places of growth, see the positive effects, and commit to writing them down by starting the sentence, "When _____ happened, it was the best thing that happened to me because of _____." Committing to this process can change the emotional charge associated with the memory, and this can be a visceral exercise in reprogramming your mind.

The Present: Take the statement you wrote about what is currently frustrating you or that you perceive as being difficult and ask yourself, "What would this look like if it was easy?" Create two columns in your journal:

It's hard because....	It's easy because.....

Sometimes we are so committed to the struggle of things being hard or frustrating that we forget to see the many ways these challenges are quite simple. I've heard from the teens I've worked with that even though this is such a simple exercise, it's effective because they've rarely focused on the aspects of the task or challenge that are simple. Instead, they are always focusing on what's hard. Giving both equal attention allows them to step into the challenge with some strength and ammunition and primes their mind for reframing things in the moment.

The Future: The final reframing tool I use I picked up from a podcast I heard years ago. It was with an athlete, an Olympic hopeful, whose dream was to be selected to compete as a member of the US rowing team. He was laser focused on his dream and every decision he made. From ordering an ice cream cone to which university he chose to study at, he asked himself one simple question, "Will this decision get me on the boat?" It's up to each one of us to define our dream and discover what our individual "boats" are, so when we are faced with a decision, we make a choice in alignment with our dreams. Every time I tell this story in my courses, each teen is then challenged to find their personal metaphor. That's the one they then use as a map to stay on path.

Beliefs

Our beliefs have been a consistent theme throughout this book. As we explored in Core Beliefs & Origins in Chapter 5, beliefs come from our practiced patterns of thinking. The brain doesn't determine what truth is, rather it accepts any thought we think habitually. Habitual thinking informs our reticular activating system to notice evidence in alignment with that belief, even if the belief is a false belief.

Imagine you were two years old, and you witnessed a scene in your family's living room as you sat on the floor and played with your blocks. Perhaps your parents were arguing. Both parents raised their voices at each other, then your father stormed out of the room and slammed the door. The door slam vibrated loudly and startled your two-year-old self, and you began to cry. Maybe you felt uneasy, unsafe, and likely scared. This emotionally jarring experience has become wired into your brain through this event anchored by the emotional charge. More than likely, your two-year-old brain created a basic meaning to the experience such as loud noises and yelling mean I'm not safe. Though you have probably forgotten this incident in your conscious mind, the first experience and likely many more throughout your life have affirmed this belief.

Fast forward to your life now. It's probable you haven't thought of this original event for years, but perhaps you've noticed you automatically become uneasy if you hear a door slam, generating a feeling of not being safe. These sorts of associations and beliefs live within your own mind, and oftentimes, we are not even aware they are there. When we are young, our brains make the connections they need in order for the world around us to make sense. Sometimes those connections get carried over into our belief system, and we may not look at or challenge them into adulthood.

I love using this next tool to help uncover some of those beliefs. A lot of our core beliefs may be from our old programming, and it is always an interesting process to uncover just what's there. When using this next tool, please don't overthink it. Don't try to discover why a particular belief exists or uncover its origin. That's not important. What is important is using the act of self-inquiry to discover your own operating system and recognizing that sometimes there are false beliefs woven through us, coloring the way we move through life.

If you find you or your teen struggling with this tool, look at the question, take a few deep breaths, close your eyes, and ask, "What do I really believe?" Remember, don't judge the answer, and it doesn't really matter if the answer is true or not.

Statement	Examples (Find your own)	Your Belief
Life, in general, is:	*good, bad, hard, a struggle, predetermined, unfair, like a box of chocolates*	
The world is:	*dangerous, unfair, filled with rules, ugly, your oyster, beautiful*	
People always:	*cheat, rip you off, are nice, act like dicks, are good*	
People don't:	*respect each other, care about other people, fear one another, help one another*	
Friends should:	*treat me with respect, care, be there, help me, support me*	
My friends always:	*disappoint me, support me, leave me, betray me*	
Family should:	*show their love, be there, support, be a safe place*	

My family always:	*judges me, makes my life difficult, loves me, helps me*	
People always treat me:	*well, horribly, fairly, based on how I treat them*	
The world owes me:	*opportunities, a living, love, nothing, everything*	
I can't:	*believe in myself, do anything right, fail*	
I always:	*get what I want, fail, make a fool out of myself, come out on top*	
I never:	*know what to do, choose the right option, fail, succeed, take risks*	
I don't deserve:	*success, love, friends, anything*	
I am meant to (do or be) in life:	*be successful, dance on stage, be famous, change the world*	

Relationships are:	*scary, stupid, unfair, terrifying, the reason for living*	
I attract into my life:	*people that are bad for me, great challenges, drama, good people, people who want to hurt me, opportunities*	
My health (or the body) is:	*powerful, strong, weak, sickly, struggling, ugly, fat*	
Money:	*comes easy, is the root to all evil, comes and goes, grows on trees*	

Fear

Let's talk about fear. We've learned about the effects fear has on the brain throughout this book. We've explored the function of the amygdala and unpacked its power to override other systems to keep us safe, conjuring up life-saving, split-second decisions to prevent us from stepping off that cliff or running head-on into traffic.

Fear can run our lives and, in some cases, ruin our lives. Fear can cause us to live with increased stress or anxiety, prompting the amygdala into a state of hyperawareness surrounding potential (real or imagined) threats. Fear can hijack normal information-processing sequences in our brains, activating our survival instincts in situations where it just might not be necessary. The amygdala, which does not have a sense of time, may be processing a threat assessment based on something that happened to you twenty years ago. As we know, those past experiences turn into thoughts, and thoughts habitually thought become beliefs.

Fearful thoughts can be just as crippling as being chased by a bear. These thoughts may produce the same reactions propelling us into fight, flight, or freeze responses. This is why I use this diagram in my practice as a cognitive tool to examine our fearful thoughts, their effects, and to pull apart the power they have in our lives.

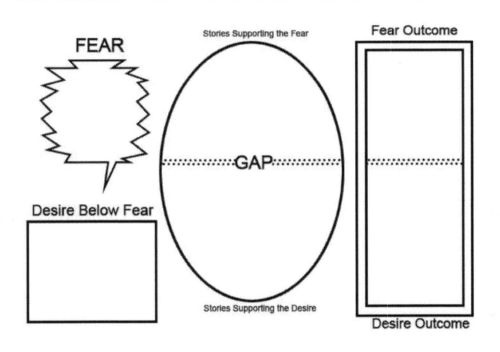

Your first job is to identify and articulate the fear you will be working with.

Fear – At the far left of the diagram, please write out the fearful thought you've identified in the area labeled "Fear."

Desire Below the Fear – Every fearful thought has a built-in desire that charges our fears. For example, you, as the parent, might have the fear that your teen won't be prepared for life. The desire below that fear would be that your teen *is* prepared for life. However, not all fears have a direct opposite desire. Take for example, you teen may fear they will never fit in. The desire below that fear might be to have a close group of friends, etc.

Fear Outcome – On the far-right corner of the page is the box labeled "Fear Outcome." Here, write out a bulleted list of at least 5 items to describe what will happen when that fear turns into a reality. For the fear, "My teen won't be prepared for life," maybe some of the fear outcomes would be:

- My teen cannot hold down a job and constantly gets fired.
- My teen resents me.
- My teen lives with me until they are 45.
- My teen doesn't figure out their passions or purpose.
- My teen is a miserable person.
- My teen doesn't talk to me.

Let yourself reveal those deep dark fears you may be too embarrassed to say out loud. Acknowledge the hidden fears that are there, even if they are a faint thought, bring it out and write it down.

Desired Outcome – Below the fear outcome is a box to add the bullet points of your desired outcome. Just as you did above, daydream, go big, and list out all the desires you have in a list format. For the desire, "My teen is prepared for life," the list might look something like this:

- My teen has great relationships in their life.
- My teen is following their dreams.
- My teen is conscious about others.
- My teen is responsible and considerate.
- My teen understands finances and budgeting.
- My teen is happy in their life.

The Gap – In the center of the diagram, there is a space called "The Gap." This is where you will add the evidence you see today which supports either the fear outcome or the desired outcome, depending on which section you are focusing on. Remember you will see, notice, and recognize lots of evidence based on where you are focusing. There will be evidence in both areas; however, the cognitive processing of both the fear and desire empowers you to make a choice where you want to place your attention.

The feedback I've gotten from this tool is that the power lies in listing out the potential outcomes on both sides. The fears feel silly, and the desires feel empowering. By using this tool, you now have accessible information to reframe the fear the moment it comes up.

Core Values

This tool is adapted from my time working in advertising and branding. Before Miro and I left on our travels, we defined what values we held dear to us, and those values helped us navigate the world. This tool can help you and your teen do the same. I've always said, we don't need rules if we are aware of our core values.

Our core values are at the root of who we are. They are what makes us tick, and they are how we process the world around us. These values are not always spoken, but the more attention we spend on defining them, the more we can choose to live in alignment with them. They can help us make decisions and define our sense of self.

The first tool I offer is a way to determine what values you are currently living. Please answer the questions below without overthinking.

What do you fill your personal space with or what are the things you like to keep around you? *Indicate at least three items that have high value to you.*	
How do you spend **your** time? *This is your free time, the time that's not managed by somebody else. What do you like to do when you are completely alone? Is it painting, dancing, etc.?*	
What energizes you? *This is the activity that you feel most alive when doing. Maybe it's playing sports, acting, or anything that gets your blood pumping.*	

What do you spend your money on? *This is your money without obligation, whatever you have earned or saved from chores and birthdays – not money spent on necessities. What is your favorite thing to treat yourself to?*	
Where in your life are you most organized or ordered? *For some people, this is how they organize their books or video game collection, the way their desk is put together, maybe even how the files are arranged on their computer.*	
Where in your life are you most disciplined and reliable? *This is the area or areas your friends and family can really count on you*	

to consistently show up and be depended upon.	
What do you spend time thinking about? *What goes through your mind when nothing else is going on? What are you planning, organizing, or fantasizing about?*	
What do you visualize? *This ties in with what you think about but is slightly different. Of those thoughts going through your head, which are the ones that you can vividly see images of?*	

What do you internally dialogue about? *This directly relates to all of the conversations we have with ourselves in the course of a day. What problems are you trying to work through or what goal are you looking to accomplish?*	
What do you want to talk to others about the most? *You feel this buildup of excitement inside of you to finally be able to have these conversations or engagements with others. These are things you are so passionate about you cannot keep them to yourself.*	

What is inspiring to you? *This could be a person, place, or thing. If there was a really great role model in your life or famous person you idolize, write down their name and figure out why. Maybe it's great art or being alone in nature. Whatever the answer is, recognizing it allows you to do more of it.*	
What are the 3 most consistent goals you've had or the 3 things you've always wanted? *Pick the three things that have been on your mind for quite some time. What have you always wanted to do, or even do more of?*	

What do you love learning about? *This can tie in with some of your other answers, or it can be completely different. When you are alone, what is it that interests you the most, something that you can never get your fill of?*	

The next step after answering these questions is to distill each of your answers into a value.

A value is defined as something (such as a principle or quality) intrinsically valuable or desirable.

An example of an answer to the question: "What do you fill your personal space with or what are the things you like to keep around you?" might be something like my artwork, my guitars, and my team sports trophies. One possible way of distilling that answer into values might look like this list of values:

- Creativity
- Expression
- Teamwork
- Perseverance
- Commitment

After you've distilled the values from your answer, look for any patterns. Finally, determine the top five values you are currently living.

Next, you may want to explore a list of values that are aspirational, meaning you are not currently living but wish to adapt. There are several ways to determine which values are aspirational to you by creating a list of values to "try on" for the week. The most straightforward way is to read through the following list of values and select the top-five values you'd aspire to live.

In the work I do with the teens, I've prepared value cards, where each teen is asked to choose the values that resonate most with them. They print out and place each card into one of three piles: Pile 1: Values I am currently living, Pile 2: Value I wish to live, and Pile 3: Values that don't resonate with me. It takes some time to move the values into the three piles, but when they are finished, they have a clear idea of what values appeal to them.

Values

Abundance - Riches; good fortune; success and bounty.	Achievement - Producing powerful desired results; accomplishment.	Adaptability - To change actions, course, or approach to doing things in order to suit a new situation; ability to learn from experience.	Wisdom - Application of knowledge in a common-sense manner; insight; good judgment.
Tradition - Long-established behavior; ongoing pattern of culture; beliefs or practices.	Trust - Confidence; reliance; safekeeping.	Truth - Authentic; candid; honest.	Simplicity - Clear; plain; straightforward; freedom from complexity.

Sobriety - Living free from addiction.	Safety - Focus on refuge, sanctuary, or shelter; freedom from risk or danger.	Resourcefulness - Creative; clever; inventive; ingenuity.	Stability - Steadfast; reliable.
Status - Prestige; position or rank showing achievement.	Success - Achieving goals; earning recognition; honors; wealth; position and rewards.	Flexibility - Ability to respond in a context appropriate emotional matter.	Being of Service - Choice to engage without expectation of reciprocation.
Dependability - Capable of being depended on; worthy of trust and reliable.	Influence - To positively impact the behavior or thinking of a person without direct control or effort; to positively impact the course of a thing, an event, or a process.	Balance - Equity; harmony; equitable distribution; A harmonious or equitable arrangement or proportion of parts or elements.	Commitment - To honor obligations; to do what I say I am going to do.
Cooperation - Working together for a common purpose or benefit.	Open Mindedness - Willing to consider new ideas and be unprejudiced.	Generosity - Gracious giving without expecting a personal return.	Authority - Persuasive force; accepted control; recognized source or

			expert on a subject.
Relationships - Companionship from fond social bonds; social connections; association with others.	Fairness - Free from bias; rational; upholding equal values.	Flexibility - Willing or open to modification or adaptation; able to manage constant change.	Harmony - Balance; good rapport; agreement among all elements.
Love - Warm emotional attachment; affection; adoration; deep caring without direct control or effort.	Financial Well-being - Able to meet financial obligation; feeling secure about the future; enjoying life.	Religion/Spirituality - Set of beliefs or practices organized around your faith.	Fun - Merry celebration; amusement; adventure; playfulness; humor.
Reliability - The quality of being trustworthy or of performing consistently well.	Good Health - Positive well-being; to include physical and mental health.	Leadership - The action of leading a group of people or an organization.	Family - A group of related people.

Freedom - Autonomy; to do as one wishes to do.	Tolerance - Open-minded; enduring.	Competition - Contest or rivalry to gain supremacy.	Beauty - Attractive; aesthetically pleasing.
Self-care - The practice of taking action to preserve or improve one's own mental and/or physical health.	Honor - Adherence to what is right, with high respect; and great esteem.	Integrity - Discipline of being ethical and moral; acting with character and honesty.	Excellence - Seeking the highest quality; commitment to the highest standard.
Effectiveness - Producing powerful desired results or intended outcomes.	Adventure - Involving an element of risk or newness; enjoying a challenge.	Inclusion - Celebrate diverse people, experiences, perspectives, and geographies; foster belonging.	Community - A feeling of fellowship with others, as a result of sharing common attitudes and interests.
Independence - Ability to make your own choices; free from outside influence.	Compassion - Selflessness; interest or care for another's welfare; desire to alleviate suffering.	Change - To make different; refine; continuous improvement.	Communication - Conveying or exchanging information clearly.

Positivity - The practice of being or tendency to be positive or optimistic in attitude.	Growth Mindset Mastery - A special level of proficiency; commitment to becoming your best self.	Peace/Tranquility - Serenity; calm; harmony; quiet.	Punctuality - Conscientious of being on time; ready; reliable; prompt.
Innovation - Creator of new ideas, creative thoughts, and new imaginations in form a of device or method.	Knowledge - Understanding gained through experience or study; information; awareness; facts.	Loyalty - Faithful allegiance; devotion.	Humor - The quality of being amusing or comic, especially as expressed in literature or speech.
Respect - A feeling of deep admiration for someone or something elicited by their abilities, qualities, or achievements.	Honesty - Genuine; straightforward; truthful.	Environmentalism - Concern about and action aimed at protecting the environment.	Perseverance - Persistence in doing something despite difficulty or delay in achieving success.
Optimism - Hopefulness and confidence about the future or the successful outcome of something.	Courage - The ability to do something that frightens one.	Innovation - A new idea or method; the next, better evolution of a device or method.	Compassion - The feeling that arises when you are confronted with another's suffering and feel motivated

			to relieve that suffering.
Happiness - Delight; joy; satisfaction; contentment; pleasure.	Power - Influence or control over people, places, or things.	Gratitude - The quality of being thankful; readiness to show appreciation for and to return kindness.	Personal Growth - Evolving of self in mind, body, spirit, or all of these.
Passion - A strong feeling of love or enthusiasm.	Creativity - The use of the imagination or original ideas, especially in the production of an artistic work.	Efficiency - The state or quality of being efficient.	Consistency - Steadfast adherence to the same principles, course, form, etc.
Perfection - The highest degree of proficiency; error-free; flawless.	Resilience - Ability to rebound or recover from loss, difficulty, failure, trauma, or disturbing experiences.	Decisiveness - Firm; resolute; taking action.	Discipline - Regimented; habit; behavior aligned with personal commitments,

Finally, after you have determined the 5 aspirational values you'd like to try on for the week, create a chart that looks like this:

Value #1	Value #2	Value #3	Value #4	Value #5	N/A

Instead of the words "Value #1," replace it with the new aspirational value you've chosen to try on for the week. Every day, in the evening, before you go to bed for one week, review your day. Write down your actions, choices, incidents, engagements, and challenges of the day under the corresponding value. Translate each incident into a single word or short phrase.

For example, if you are trying on the value "tolerance" as Value #1, recognize that when your sister said that unkind thing to you today, you didn't snap back at her. That would be living the value of "tolerance." Write her name or a short phrase to represent that incident in column 1.

If the day's incidents, challenges, or decisions don't fall under any of those values, place it in the column marked "N/A" (not applicable). Keep a record for one week, reviewing your day each night. The goal of this exercise is to have more entries each night in the five values columns than in the N/A column. Normally, after the first day, more of the day's incidents and your reaction to them tend to fall within the five values categories. It's exciting to see the changes!

After a week, decide if this new aspirational value should be transformed into one of your core values. You will find when you bring focus to your values, they will naturally assist you to make choices, decisions, and actions that are in alignment with the values you embrace. It's empowering!

Worldviews

The understanding of worldviews is important in any context, not just raising teens. But to my surprise, many families I've worked with, who do not travel, have never considered this important aspect of being in the world.

Worldviews focus on our shared perspectives, viewpoints, and norms based on many influences, including culture. It is the foundation for a belief system in which we see and explain the world. Worldviews serve as a lens through which the world is interpreted, which influences one's perspective, values, and actions. In most cases, the belief systems we are born into are influenced by the dominant social norms from within our culture.

Think of it from this perspective, it is almost impossible for a fish to differentiate the things he sees in his path of vision without the distortion caused by light refracting on the water surrounding him. The nature of his reality is seeing his world through water; there is no other way.

Consider some of the factors that are omnipresent for you. In my case, one factor was being born in the US. By default, I had an "American-centric" view of the world, which wasn't observable in my perception until I left the US.

Think about getting your vision tested as a metaphor. A visit to the optometrist always includes interacting with a machine called a phoropter. Looking through this device, the optometrist inserts different lenses and relies on your feedback to let them know which lens or lens combination allows you to see the clearest. Worldviews are very much like that machine. The lenses filter the way we see the world.

I recall thinking, as a child growing up in California, that it had to be the best place in the world to live. It was the only place I knew, but it seemed perfect compared to my nonexistent knowledge of anywhere else. Now that I haven't lived in California in over thirteen years and have traveled to many other new and exciting places, I can't believe I ever once had that perspective. It is difficult to be reflective about things when you are in the middle of living them. While everyone is different and needs to find the tools and experiences that work for them, travel is what helped me get crystal clear about the worldviews coloring my life.

The truth about worldviews is that although we do not often see the actual lens itself (like how the fish doesn't see the water), we see the world through those lenses. They are the primary influence contributing to how we see the world.

But culture is not the only influence that colors our worldviews. There are other external factors we are born into such as our family's race, social-economic status, political affiliations, religion, and specific geographical location. Then our individual identities add to the many lenses already in place like age, gender, and personal experiences.

Another component that adds to a person's worldview is idealism(s). There are a lot of identity politics currently surrounding these "isms," and people are absorbing a whole set of worldviews without reflecting to see if they are in alignment with who they really are (or their values). This is not a political conversation, but an invitation to dig deep and see what we might be getting influenced by. First, ask if each individual part and piece is in alignment with what you truly believe. Making adjustments makes us more developed as humans. As we've discussed, there is no such thing as truth in the brain. It only has belief systems, and there is no difference between truth and lies.

Teens can be influenced by what they feel they are supposed to be or do in life, which is a natural product of their own internalization. The American-centric worldview is that teens need to grow up after they graduate high school, go to college, and get a good job. The timing of all of that happening by eighteen may not be possible for every teen due to their own schedule or the state of the world. Because we impose this on them, they wind up feeling pressured into picking a major and finding a job. The world is set up to pigeonhole teens in the worst possible way. When parents don't challenge this belief, they are allowing their kids to go along with this as their dominant belief, which doesn't serve teens at all. Some teens may know exactly what they want to do at this stage, but most will not, and they should be given the time to figure it out.

Worldviews help to provide us with answers to the big questions. As an exercise, answer the questions below with full awareness of how your worldview impacts your answers.

Exploring Worldviews as a Tool

Understanding that worldviews are lenses that color how we see the world and that all our worldviews are unique. Use the questions below to help you identify yours.

Identifying Your Unique Lenses

Age:	
Gender Identity:	

Sexual Orientation:	
Religion / Spiritual Beliefs:	
Family Structure:	
Ethnicity:	
Nationality:	
Class / Economic Status:	
Philosophical Ideals:	
Education:	

Location:	
Political Views:	
Cultural Traditions & Practices:	
Family Culture / Values:	
Language:	
Diet:	
Entertainment Preferences:	
Social Cliques:	

Physical Appearance:	
Mental Health Status:	
Physical Health Status:	
Relationship(s) Status:	
Transformational Personal Experiences:	
Core Values:	

Recognize the effort it took to define all those things. Recognize that no one else could have answered these questions exactly as you did. Your perspective and worldview are unique. Now, run a big world issue through this lens. Ask yourself any **big** question. One example might be, "How can we achieve world peace?"

Your answer will be the summation of all your answers above. If you change one or a dozen of those answers, the response to the big question will change.

The idea is to realize there is no right or wrong way to answer any question, but recognize that those who have different worldviews based on differing answers to the questions above have valuable perspectives too.

In my course, I pair up teens and have them co-create characters by answering the questions above. Then we create circumstances, put the characters in, and explore how and why they'd react, respond, and act differently based on their unique worldview. It's a powerful eye-opener, and at the end of the exercise, every teen develops deeper compassion for a diversity of worldviews.

Once your teen has fully grasped the concept of worldviews, ask them these more philosophical questions to consider:

How did we get here?	
Why are we here?	
Who am I?	
Where are we going?	

Who's in charge?	
What is truth?	
What is right?	
What is wrong?	
Am I living a good life?	

Passions & Purpose

I love this topic so much and have run entire courses specifically helping adolescents define their passions and purpose. Witnessing a teen discover a purpose is one of the most rewarding experiences ever! Although I'm only including a few tools here, they will kickstart a valuable lifelong journey.

Before a teen can do the work around discovering their passions and purpose, it's a good idea to identify what beliefs they hold in order to explore this topic in a way that makes sense to them.

Choose which statement most resonates with you (your teen):

1. You think that no one actually has an "official life purpose," and you just move through life as it comes, making your own choices based on opportunities.
2. You believe you know or sense exactly what your life purpose is. and you work towards it every day.
3. Everyone is born with a life purpose or reason for being here, but you haven't yet discovered what yours is.
4. None of the above, write your belief here:_____.

Create a dialogue around their answer and explore what this really means to them and how their beliefs can potentially impact their future.

Here are two follow-up questions to explore with your teen. Read both, and ask your teen to explore which statement feels truer to them:

1. Predetermination: Do you believe you are born with a predetermined life purpose, which includes gifts, talents, and abilities that you are meant to use? Is this a responsibility you have to the world?
2. Free will: Do you believe life is a journey to discover your life purpose, develop your gifts, talents, and abilities, and choose how to use them as you see fit?

Explore this a little deeper. Ask this question addressing natural born talents, "When a person is born with a natural talent for something (musical ability, aptitude in math, charismatic speaker, etc.), do you believe you are obligated to use that talent in some way?"

I've often heard teens confess that their parents believe they have a natural ability at something (athlete, painter, scientist, etc.) and hear from their parents that they feel it's a "waste" not to use their natural ability. Is this how you feel as a parent? Is this the message or pressure your teen gets from you? This is something to unpack together and discuss.

Again, there is no right or wrong way to answer these questions, but creating dialogue around this topic will help your teen articulate their feelings better and help you as the facilitator to unpack and apply the following tools in a way that best supports them.

What is passion? Many teens can tap into what that means for them by recognizing what lights them up and makes them come alive. Some teens have no idea what they are passionate about, and some are born knowing their passions.

What is purpose? Purpose goes just a little deeper than passion. It's that motivation to look at the bigger picture, to recognize passion as the fuel to serve ourselves, others, and the world around us.

Before one can discover their true life purpose, they need to uncover some clues. Namely, things they are good at, feel passionate about, love to do, and are important to them. The tool below will help your teens uncover their passions and purpose.

Under each column, create a bulleted list with at least ten short answers. Push yourself to expand, explore, and discover answers that may be buried deep inside. After all, information about your passion and purpose are found inside each one of us.

Activities I love to do:	Topics or subjects I'm passionate about:	Things I'm naturally good at:	Things that are important to me (world, social, and human issues, outside of me):

After filling out the tool above, reflect on which answers were easy to access and which were difficult to define. Were there any answers that surprised you? Take another look at the worksheet. Do you see any connections or patterns between the items you listed? You may not yet have a full picture, rather a handful of puzzle pieces, and you can see they could fit together but you're not sure how.

Let's frame this information through a powerful metaphor. Imagine that you are preparing to take a journey. Your first task should be to define your destination. You may need to find a large map so you can see all the possible routes. What are the most important things you need to make this journey successful? Finally, select how you'll travel, which mode of transportation you'll use and which type of fuel you need to power it.

Within this metaphor, think of your life purpose like the journey. Think of the things you love doing as the vehicle that will get you there. Think of your natural talents as a map that shows you the routes to your destination. The things that are important to your journey are translated into the destination. And what fuels the vehicle? Well, that's your passion.

Why do we need to live our life with purpose?

"Purpose is the fuel that wakes me up every single day. Without purpose, I just go on autopilot, I don't think anymore. I really need it as guidance in my life."

~ Luc van Hoeckel, Director of Social Impact at Adidas and Co-Founder of Super Local

Living with purpose helps us naturally find balance in our lives, leading to long-term satisfaction, fulfillment, and, dare I say, happiness. Broadly speaking, having a sense of purpose means we have a road map to direct us towards a particular destination. For some, that means creating a structure with concrete goals in mind. For others, that means knowing there's a direction and the details are yet to be defined. While life provides ups and downs, having purpose in life can contribute to greater states of motivation and long-term happiness.

The last tool I'll share in this section is a powerful tool I assign the adolescents in my courses to use. This is often one of their favorite challenges, and teens consistently report they've uncovered some wonderful surprises.

Ask your teen to select at least three people around them: family, friends, relatives, teachers, mentors, parents, and peers. Those around us often find it easier to see things in us that we may have a difficult time seeing in ourselves. We've all got blind spots after all. Ask your teen to conduct their interviews in person if they can and write out the answers. If in-person interviews are not possible, they can also send them the questions and ask them to return their answers via email or other messaging apps. Here are the questions to ask:

1. What do you think I was born to do?
2. What do you think I am really good at?
3. What skills do you see in me that might be underused at this time?
4. What career path would you recommend for me?
5. What are the things you think I have expertise in?
6. What am I doing when you perceive me as being the happiest?

After you've received the answers from all your interviews, review them and look for patterns. Ask your teen to journal these questions:

How do I feel about these answers?
What new discoveries did I make about myself?
What surprised me?
What things about me were confirmed?
What patterns are coming up in all the answers?
According to all the work I've done around this topic, my life purpose should be defined as what?

People-Pleasing & Boundaries

People-pleasing is a trait many parents subconsciously expect of their children. Especially when our kids are young, parents oftentimes just expect their kids to happily go along with whatever is most convenient for the family. Put on your shoes, hug your grandma, say "thank you," and wash your dirty cereal bowl. These all might be reasonable requests, but the expectation that our kids do them is associated with consequences. The consequence of not complying is less important than the consequence of children learning that pleasing others is an important skill they need in order to get along in life.

To be clear, there is no judgment here. We were all raised with these sorts of expectations, and there is certainly no implication that this is right or wrong. I'm simply stating that within our culture, we all have been trained to some extent to please someone else over our own needs or desires. It's the degree to which we continue this throughout our life that is critical here.

In this next tool, ask your teen to rate from 0 to 10 the degree in which this answer is true for them, 10 being the truest and 0 representing not true at all. If you answered with a number of 1 or over (not 0), write into the notes section the last time this incident occurred in your life.

Question:	Rate 0 to 10	Notes:
I generally agree with people to avoid conflict.		
I have a hard time saying "no" to people?		
When I help others, I do it out of obligation and oftentimes feel resentment.		
I am always really hard on myself, and when I make mistakes, I am super critical of myself.		
I strive for perfection in most things I do.		

I often tell people I am ok when I am not actually ok.		

Add up your score. If you scored anything above the number 30, you have some tendency to people-please.

I have to admit, I am a recovering people pleaser. There are varying viewpoints on whether this is a good or bad thing, but at the core, it is neither. It is, however, something that must be kept in balance by maintaining personal boundaries. Once we allow the needs of others to take priority over our own, we tread on dangerous territory.

Think about your boundaries like the hurdles that track runners have to leap over. Each one of those hurdles is an integral piece of helping to keep the balance between making others happy and living our own truth. When you constantly put the needs of others first at your own expense, it is like laying all those hurdles down for them to be walked all over. That is not balanced.

In this next tool, you'll need to use one of the examples from the "Notes" section in the worksheet above. You can use this tool with **every example** from the Notes section if you have the patience.

Recent people-pleasing incident:	Boundary crossed:	Boundary I am now committing to:
My mom asked if I was ok, I was not. I was feeling depressed but I said I was fine.	*I did not speak my truth.*	*I speak my truth.*
I agreed to help my friend with her project, but I didn't really have the time (or want to do it).	*I prioritized someone else's needs over mine.*	*I prioritize my needs and desires first.*

Goals & Accountability

Professional athletes set countless goals in the course of a day, week, or month, and they use coaches and trainers to be accountable to. When they don't meet their goals, this allows their trainers to identify where the breakdown happened and create a strategy to get them back on track. As a parent, we can support our teens in much of the same way, as long as we do this with the request of our teens and within the scope of partnership.

Creating goals is one of the best tools we have to hold ourselves accountable. We can utilize the skills we learned surrounding milestones and think about our passions and purpose to drive goals. And let's not forget, as we achieve our goals, we are releasing dopamine, which feels good and keeps us on track.

You can teach goals or accountability without experiencing it. In my course, I challenge the teens to create and execute a project. I find this to be one of the best ways to help facilitate goal setting and accountability, and you can do the same with your teen if they consent. Your role in the project will be as an accountability partner. Agree to regular check-ins and facilitate whatever support they may need. The goal of partnering with them on a project is to foster a deeper connection, not to step into the role of the teacher or disciplinarian. Remember, failure on a project provides just as much learning as a successful project execution.

Here are questions to help your teen brainstorm their project:

What would you do if you were guaranteed success (not capable of failing)?	
What would you do if you had a superpower?	
What would you do if you had no fear?	
What would give you great joy upon completion?	
What makes you nervous? You know you want to do it, but you have fear or hesitation because you might fail.	
What would you do if money and time were not an issue?	
What kind of mentor would you need in order to get your project finished?	

Once your teen has an idea of their project, define the project details here:

Describe your project in one paragraph:
What is your project objective? *(Example: I want to design a 30-day inspirational calendar for my friends using inspirational quotes from contemporary music.)*
When your project is complete, how will you know it was successful?

Describe your final project deliverable:
(Example: presentation, website, video, piece of art, book, creative writing, etc.)

Next, use the chart below to help organize this project into 4 distinct steps or phases:

Describe the process in step 1:	
Define the deliverable at the end of step 1 needed to move on to the next step:	
Date to be completed:	
Notes:	

Describe the process in step 2:	
Define the deliverable at the end of step 2 needed to move on to the next step:	
Date to be completed:	
Notes:	
Describe the process in step 3:	

Define the deliverable at the end of step 3 needed to move on to the next step:	
Date to be completed:	
Notes:	
Describe the process in step 4:	
Define the deliverable at the end of step 4 which should be the finished project:	

Date to be completed:	
Notes:	

There are many more complex formulas to map out project development using project management tools, but the simplified format above creates enough awareness of what deliverables are, how they lead into the next phase, and committing to dates for delivery.

Conflict Resolution

Learning conflict resolution skills is so important at any stage of life. I teach the principles of Nonviolent Communication (NVC) in my courses, but here we are going to focus on one of my favorite tools called Thomas-Kilmann Conflict Mode Instrument (TKI). This tool has been used successfully for more than 30 years to help groups in a variety of settings understand how different conflict styles affect personal and group dynamics. This tool is commonly used in the workplace for managing teams, but I like to use this tool with teens because it's simple to understand and use. We have lots of fun using the different styles to role-play different situations to really understand what they feel like. There are lots of videos explaining this tool online, so if you're interested, do a quick search.

Here's the TKI tool a nutshell:

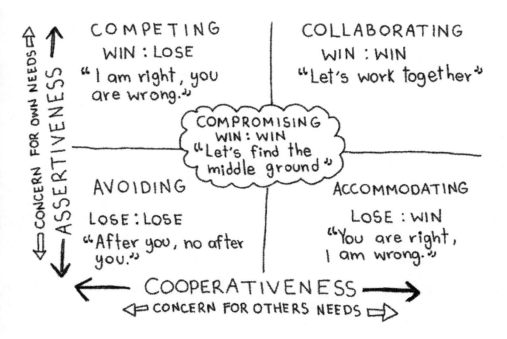

There are two main axes that each of the styles of resolution lay on: assertiveness and cooperation. Each of the five conflict resolution styles integrate different degrees of both.

Competing: In the top left of the chart, we have competing as a solution, which is high on assertiveness and low on cooperation. One of the traits of competing is being assertive and uncooperative with the opposing party. However, this strategy is not all bad, being that this strategy is most appropriate when a speedy resolution is needed and the two parties have disproportionate positions of power. It is also a good choice to use this mode when someone must make a tough choice.

Avoiding: Avoiding is the most passive form of conflict resolution, low on cooperativeness and assertiveness. Ideally, we should face conflicts head-on; however, there are some situations where confrontation is best avoided.

Or, you may encounter a conflict that is so trivial, it is simply not worth your time.

The avoiding approach involves staying clear of the conflict, withholding one's views and opinions, and simply not engaging. People may choose this approach when the personal cost of confrontation may be far greater than the cost of living with the conflict. To be clear, avoiding does not actually resolve the conflict. It just buries it below the surface and may potentially lead to future problems.

Accommodating: The accommodating approach strives to call a truce in order to resolve the conflict. However, in order to accommodate, one or the other is giving up their position, stance or side. Choosing this approach may be worthwhile in situations when you feel the conflict is a total waste of your time.

With this approach, you are required to be high in cooperativeness and low in assertiveness, which means your priority is making the other party happy.

Collaborating: This approach is most effective when both parties in the conflict are really on the same page or have the same goal or outcome in mind. Most feel this is an ideal solution, but it can only happen when both parties are sensible, hold similar positions of authority, and are ready to be cooperative.

In order to collaborate, typically, the first step is engaging in a detailed discussion in order to understand each other's viewpoints. The goal of collaboration is to reach a solution where both parties benefit.

Compromising: Finally, at the center of the Thomas Kilmann Conflict Mode Instrument is compromising, a point where moderate assertiveness and moderate cooperativeness are required. In certain situations, the best choice may be compromised in order to come to a faster solution when both parties don't really have the time to collaborate. There may also be some situations where both parties won't budge on their stance, and by choosing to compromise, both parties get to say what their position is and what they are willing to do. This option is really a mixed bag: both win, both lose.

Shadow Work

During the shadow workshops I facilitate in my mentorship programs, I introduce shadow work as simply befriending the parts of ourselves we've deemed unworthy or unlovable. However, diving into our shadows, healing our inner child, and integrating the unloved parts of ourselves can be a lifelong process. Introducing this concept to adolescents can help them start to love themselves in ways they hadn't even imagined. But this work isn't for the faint of heart.

I've designed and facilitated intensive 30-day shadow workshops for adults, but in this section, I'm sharing with you a couple of the basic tools I use with teens in order to facilitate an introduction to their darker sides. Conversations about shame and our unloved parts are not easy, so when I work with teens, I invite them to do the work on paper and ask questions but take time to sit with the things they uncover without sharing. Knowing they have support to do this work is important.

Overall, the main purpose of doing shadow work is to start to integrate all the parts of ourselves we've disowned, create a relationship with our own shame, and recognize when shame is controlling our behavior. In those moments when the darkness threatens to consume us, shadow work helps us to shine a light on it and to expose it to ourselves, removing much of its power.

Integrating the shadow into one's consciousness requires brutal objectivity in observation of one's own impulses and triggers. Integration of the shadow is hard; almost no one ever truly achieves completion. It requires transparent honesty and courage to reveal the unaccepted and unloved parts of oneself.

To begin facing your shadow is to withdraw your projections from the external world and then integrate these elements of your personality into conscious awareness. In other words, to face your shadow is to acknowledge your potential for darkness, then rather than avoiding it because it detests you, bring it into the light of day and take ownership of it.

In order to effectively participate in shadow work, we must invite in the feelings of being uncomfortable.

The first tool I use with teens is a powerful one. Using the table below, I ask teens to write a bullet-point list of the qualities, behaviors, attributes, or traits that trigger or annoy them from their parents. One side indicates those of their mother or a maternal figure, and the other is designed for those of their father or paternal figure.

Mother (Material Figure)	Father (Paternal Figure)

I usually ask them to find ten traits of each and give examples, such as, "I hate it when my mother tries to control me," or "I get triggered when my father is distant." They should write out the traits, attributes, habits, and behaviors, both large and small, whatever they can think of, by being brutally honest. (Sorry parents.)

Once the list is finished, I invite them to see which item on the list is most charged. That will be the one they'll work with in the next tool.
After looking over the list, I ask the teens to thank their parents (maternal and paternal figures) for shining light on the shadows the teens have inside of them. The qualities, behaviors, attributes, or traits from our parents that trigger us are not about our parents at all; they are about the qualities, behaviors, attributes, or traits we've embodied and rejected inside of ourselves.

It's true, many of our shadow parts come from our childhood, revealed to us through our caregivers, but they can also derive from a variety of other sources and experiences, including our individual worldviews, beliefs, preferences, and traumas.

Spectrum Tool

If two things are on two sides of the same coin or on opposite sides of the same coin, they are closely related to each other and cannot be separated, even though they seem to be completely different. Each person will have to determine their opposites as there is not a single formal guideline to refer to.

For example, some people feel that love and hate are opposite sides of the same coin. Others feel love and fear are opposites. It will depend on your perception, your belief system, and how you identify with that specific emotion or experience. This is all based on your personal perception of that feeling.

The tool below strives to support a deeper understanding of our shadows and when they are alive in our experiences. To facilitate this, start by having your teen write the shadow emotion at the far left line and the opposite emotion at the far right line. Then, fill in the spectrum of emotions, or gradations, of feelings.

Shadow

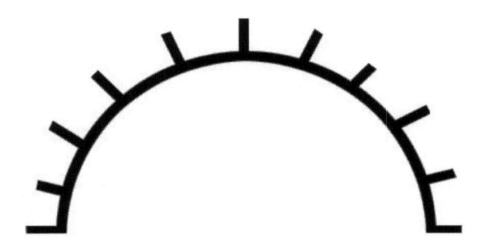

Why is this tool important?

A common misconception around shadow work is that the shadows are always the negative aspects of ourselves we have rejected, denied, suppressed, or disowned. But, in fact, there are both positive and negative shadows that are equally important to uncover.

A positive shadow might be more easily understood through my personal story. When I was young, I believed I was capable, resourceful, and confident, but I never had reinforcement in that belief because I was never very obedient. Because of my disobedience, I was not trusted nor was I raised with a sense of sovereignty; therefore, my inner sense of confidence and capability was rejected.

Over time, I began to reject those positive qualities in myself. For many years, I thought I had to choose between being myself, confident and capable, which turned into fierce independence, or being obedient, which in my mind was equal to being loved and accepted.

As an adult, I felt the independent self I had become was unlovable and often suppressed that to step into a caretaker role (archetype), becoming selfless and submissive in order to be lovable. In my adult relationships, I always had inner conflicts between who I felt I really was and who I needed to be in order to be loved. Much of these relationships were filled with pain because I felt internally divided. Once I resolved that, discovering the confident, capable, and independent part of myself I had suppressed was actually lovable, I started to integrate the shadow beliefs.

So for me, the confident, capable, and independent would be one side of the spectrum. The other side would be selfless, submissive, and caretaking, which are not complete opposites, but how my mind perceived it.

While shadows are the internalized parts of ourselves in the darkness, which we unconsciously suppress, projection is the externalization (sending out) of the shadow aspects, such as negative or positive desires, feelings, or ideas we are not aware of having. When we project our shadows onto others, we are trying to cope with aspects of ourselves we have not yet assimilated or integrated into our consciousness. Shadow projection leads to judgment and oftentimes triggers us to no end. Watch out for these reactions; they are likely your unconscious mind telling you it's time to dig deeper into your own shadows.

Of course, shadow work is much more complex than just these tools and the overview I provided. This was meant to be an introduction to the concept of helping your teens to become aware of their shadows. If you wish to pursue this topic further, I've listed some of my favorite resources in the Suggested Reading section at the end of this book.

Self-Regulation

The last tool I want to share is inspired and adapted from the book *Self-Compassion for Teens* by Lee-Ann Gray, PhD. Her book is filled with amazing tools focused on self-compassion. I find this an effective tool for self-regulation, and I love facilitating this tool in my practice. I've used this tool both in person and through zoom; both can be equally effective. Your job as the facilitator is to lead the experience, and part of that is setting an environment that's safe, private, and relaxing.

Learning to use tools like this to self-regulate helps us to ground ourselves, let go of our worries and stresses, and become fully embodied. Some may consider this to be a guided meditation, but I like to simply call it a self-regulation tool, which removes any preconceived notions people have about meditating.

Invite your teen to find a comfortable place to sit or even lie down, turn off bright lights in the room, and if your teen responds to it, add some relaxing background music. Use these prompts as a guide to narrate an experience. Please interpret each prompt into your own words and trust you are facilitating an amazing tool.

Body Scan & Grounding Tool:

> Take three deep breaths, inhale and exhale, filling up your belly and emptying it out with each exhale.
>
> Follow the air in as it enters your nose and travels through your lungs, filling your belly.
>
> Focus your attention on the flow of air, in and out, in and out, with each exhale and inhale.
>
> Notice when you feel present in your body.

Bring your attention to your spine, notice the length, starting from the top of your head, traveling down to the tailbone.

Imagine your tailbone is extending from your body.

Now, see the extended tailbone as folding and twisting into a small loop, from just outside of your spine to between the top of your legs.

Now, imagine a cord coming up from the earth. Notice it's thickness, weight, color, and width.

In your mind, connect this cord to the loop between your legs, right at the base of your spine.

Once the cord is connected to the loop, notice the cord looping around, creating a knot, tightly fastened to the loop, merging and closing the circle.

Now, notice the cord dropping down into the earth, burrowing its way through the planet, through all the layers below us.

In your mind's eye, follow the cord connected to your tailbone, traveling down into the depths of the earth.

See the cord deeper and deeper, finally coming to the core of the earth, where there is a massive bright ball of glowing reddish and golden energy.

See the cord wrapping around the core, becoming fused together.

Exhale deeply, knowing you are plugged into Mother Earth's power grid.

Feel the love and support she is sending you back up through the cord, sending you sustenance for life.

Feel the receiving of this gift, flowing from the core into your body.

Imagine all your negative thoughts, anxieties, and fears flushing out of your body through your grounding cord.

See these things traveling down the cord toward the core of the planet.

Imagine Mother Earth accepting and welcoming your offering, as a sacred gift, as powerful energy that she will transmute into that awesome ball of energy located at the center.

Feel the exchange of energy for a few more inhales and exhales, taking her love into your body, flushing out your unwanted negativity.

After a few breaths, move your attention back on your body. Start with scanning how you are feeling from the top of your head down to your toes. Check in with each and every body part. Notice if there is any tension. If you find any tension, send it down the cord like a feeding tube into the center of the earth as your sacred offering.

Continue scanning your body, check your head, face, eyes, mouth, neck, shoulders, chest, arms, legs and feet. If there are any sensations in parts of your body, just notice them without judgment.

Focus your attention now on the space inside your body. Imagine your body as a hollow vessel being filled with rich nourishing oxygen, mixing with the powerful golden energy being sent up from the core of the earth.

Breathe into your body, and with each breath, push that oxygen into your cells.

Allow this process to continue for a few moments.

When you are ready, bring your focus back into the room and open your eyes

When you are both ready, facilitate a reflection. Ask your teen questions like: How are you feeling? What it was like to be grounded to the earth? How did it feel to dispel negative thoughts, anxieties, or feelings? How did it feel to receive so much love? How did your body feel when it was being energized by oxygen and replenished with the energy of the earth?

All these practices are an act of self-compassion, which helps to regulate and calm the nervous system.

Chapter 10: Final Thoughts

Why Mentoring

I think it is fair to say that every parent wants their child to be prepared for life, to feel confident and live with value and purpose. But I think the greatest wish we have for our teens is that we want them to be happy and to be prepared for whatever life brings them. The true path to happiness can be found through an inward journey. With the help of tools, the support of people around them who truly care, and growing up in an environment where they are seen, heard, and understood, we can set our teens up to succeed.

When our teens are struggling, we often struggle too. In a time of tremendous change, teens are not always sure how to navigate a new landscape. Many times, they feel as overwhelmed and frustrated as their parents do. As parents, frequently we have blinkers on, hyper-focusing on the struggle as anger, withdrawal, rebellion, depression, self-harm, self-sabotage, or anxiety. These behaviors can leave us dumbfounded, watching our teens use the only coping skills at their disposal. At times, our teens' behaviors can be so all-encompassing, filling the family space, and not leaving room for much else.

As parents, we carry the weight of these challenges in our hearts. Sometimes, we are just too close to be an emotionally-neutral guide or mentor for our teens. Sometimes, our teens are unshakable and know their parents just can't support them in this way. Please, don't take this personally. Trust me, it's easy for us to feel rejected, frustrated, and helpless, as we watch our teens struggle to find their own way.

But there are options.

According to a scientific study published in 2011 called "Supportive Non-Parental Adults and Adolescent Psychosocial Functioning: Using Social Support as a Theoretical Framework" by E. M. Sterrett, D. J. Jones, L. G. McKee, and C. Kincaid, mentoring by a nonparental adult can provide effective support in the areas of youth psychosocial functioning, academic functioning, self-esteem, and behavioral and emotional challenges.

According to the study, most adolescents have the presence of a significant nonparental adult in their lives, and report their presence influences them in unique ways. For example, adolescents feel that nonparental adults are able to offer resources their peers are unable to, provide advice based on experience, and be objective about issues that matter most to them like relationships, sexual activity, experimentation with drinking or drugs, etc. Adolescents also report it's easier for them to share things they would not tell their parents for fear of embarrassment or punishment.

Teens have so many stressors and a world of expectations placed on them by society, family, peers, surrounding culture, and even by themselves. Most teens don't recognize these stressors, which often leads to negative habitual thinking. Research concludes that what teens need are meaningful connections in their lives and mentoring from nonparental adults.

Mentoring has also been linked in studies to social-emotional development benefits, improvements in youth and parental relationships, and better prospects for their future.

According to the journal article, "Mentoring: A Promising Strategy for Youth Development," the benefits adolescents receive as a result of having a mentor are:

- Increased self-esteem
- A sense of accomplishment
- Creation of new healthy networks
- Insight into their own development (childhood, adolescence, and young adulthood)
- Increased patience
- Compassion for self and others

Mentoring helps youth move through challenging times, navigate major life transitions, deal with stress at home, and transition into adulthood. Matching your adolescents with a mentor is a great option, even if your teen isn't struggling at the moment. Supportive and healthy relationships formed between mentors and mentees are beneficial both immediate and long-term. Mentoring empowers your teen by looking at what's active in their lives right now, without judgment or expectations. In my mentoring practice, I've witnessed teens thrive by forming meaningful relationships, where being seen, heard, and understood are at the foundation. Teens with mentors have more self-confidence, self-esteem, and can create big goals for themselves.

"Self-love and being at peace with yourself is so important and I learned so much about how to get better every time I work with Lanie."
~ Dani Helper, Teen

If you decide to seek a mentor for your teen, find someone who truly partners with each teen to facilitate self-discovery. In my practice, I do just that.

Transformative Mentoring for Teens (https://transformativementoringforteens.com) is a supported experiential journey into self through deep self-inquiry by utilizing powerful tools designed to transform your teen into a happy, confident, and self-actualized adult.

Is Coaching or Mentoring the Same as Therapy?

No, it is not!

Coaches and mentors do NOT diagnose teens. They focus on where the teen is now and help them to move forward to where they want to be. Mentoring does not focus on the past or past events. Mentoring is NOT therapy or psychological help, and if your teen is suffering from mental health issues, you should first speak to your doctor or therapist. However, mentoring does work in perfect harmony with therapy, mental health counseling, and cognitive behavioral therapy, which we'll explore a little later on in this chapter.

Idealism

Idealism is such an integral part of the adolescent experience. This is prompted by developmental changes in the brain as well as social influences. As the capacity of the teen's brain increases throughout adolescence so does the ability for abstract thinking. As adolescents move through different developmental stages, their relationship to idealism also changes. For example, early adolescence comes with heightened emotional capacity while the ability for logical reasoning is still developing a little later in their teen years. Younger teens are able to see the world in a new way based on their developing capacity for abstract thinking which can create an emotionally driven idealistic response to how the world should be. It's not until sometime in their early twenties that adolescents develop the ability to analyze their worldviews logically. It's actually all in perfect order.

My idealism brought me to punk rock, which ignited my inner spirit of challenging authority. Later in my adolescence, my idealism brought me to be active in human rights and anti-war movements. Young people undeniably drive social change, and idealism is the force behind that.

Adolescents do not have the worldly experience most adults do simply because of the number of years they've been on the planet. But in general, these are the years we most identify with movements, politics, and particular worldviews that align with our core values such as equality, environmental issues, BLM, political activism, etc. There are times when teens can become blinded by the actual application of the concept and have a hard time seeing past the idealism.

As parents, we need to be supportive and honor the fact that idealism plays an important role in human evolution, even if we do not agree with the stances our teens are taking. I've seen many families become split because of differing political viewpoints among parents and teens. Instead of the parents just accepting their child's idealistic stance, it becomes a source of contention and frustration.

If we've learned anything to this point, we know each and every one of us has a different way of seeing the world based on so many contributing factors. If you are struggling to connect with your adolescent because of different opinions, please do whatever you can to be supportive and understanding and manage your own reactions. One place you can connect with your teen, without engaging in a direct conflict about the topic, is to talk about the values from which the idealistic stances stem from. That's usually a beautiful and relational place to connect.

Here's a little secret about me in my family. Miro and I have two very different political viewpoints. Although we constantly engage in wonderfully heated explorations of the merits of both of our stances, they are always respectful and kind. I love that he has a different viewpoint than I do, and I, as a parent of an adolescent, know I've raised a freethinking, confident, and independent human. That's my wish for every teen. I love every opportunity to connect with him in the spaces that are truly uncomfortable.

This decade has brought us a divided world (politically, socially, medically) and a culture of extreme black-and-white, right-or-wrong thinking. By not making anyone's idealism wrong, we can create spaces for connection and kindness. The first place we need to practice this is in our own families.

Remember, always choose connection.

If your adolescent's idealism is really frustrating you, reframe it in this way: a different perspective in your household makes your home richer and more diverse. Change will continue to help us grow as a species.

Sovereignty, Autonomy & Consent

This section may feel a little radical for some, but I urge you to continue reading with an open mind.

Most of us don't often think about sovereignty, autonomy, and consent as core fundamentals relating to parenting. Yet, these areas have a significant impact on an adolescent's life, and I feel it's important to take a moment to unpack these concepts. Let's begin by defining each of these terms:

Sovereignty: independent authority and the right to govern itself
Autonomy: the state of existing or acting separately from others
Consent: giving permission for something to happen or be done

Although these topics may sound scary while thinking about raising a teen, as we've discovered in Chapter 6, the adolescent brain is wired to seek out greater independence. Understanding these topics, creating dialogue around them in your family, and integrating them into your parenting will support greater partnership in your family and greater mental health all around. Additionally, there is a huge advantage to having the language to talk about independence with your teen and explore the dynamics of accountability, responsibility, and support. Sounds like a win-win!

Sovereignty is a topic I have often discussed within my own family and within the context of the work I do with teens. Sovereignty should be explored through the lenses of these three domains:

- Sovereignty of self - both from a physical & thought level
- Sovereignty within relationships - how to support autonomy and how to respect consent
- Sovereignty within and without the systems - we consent to engage in

As you can see, all these concepts are bound together, reliant upon one another to be effective. But it does take tremendous effort to live with sovereignty in your family unit, especially with so many other things going on.

My greatest work surrounding sovereignty is within the domain of the mind. I support parents and teens by using tools to help them consciously deprogram their limiting beliefs, fearful patterns, and habitual thinking.

Integrating the fundamentals of sovereignty into our parenting can empower us to create greater partnerships with our families.

Consent is the permission of what you can or cannot do with the body or in the presence of another individual. An example of this could be speaking up about activities that are offensive, like off-colored jokes, making it known that consent is not given for that to happen in your presence. This can also be related to the way a parent might always force a child to kiss a relative they didn't want to or not being allowed to have a certain hairstyle because the parent doesn't approve. This tells the child they have no say and their bodily self is not really theirs. It is so important to realize this because a bad relationship with bodily autonomy, when it comes to consent, increases the chance they will allow others to violate them more than they might have consented to if they had more control of their body.

These consent issues also play into bedtimes and food choices. Parents have a tough time allowing their teens to go to sleep when they want. The longer it takes the teen to have control over bedtime, the longer the period where they are going to abuse it when they finally do have that control. Allowing a teen to self-regulate takes patience and time.

The same goes with food. If you are still telling your teen to clean their plate and eat all their vegetables, what are you telling them about their own body? If they eat ice cream for dinner for a week, eventually they will realize they are not getting the nutrients they need. Partnering with them to explore natural consequences is your job. Self-regulation is something we all need to find, but this is an inside job. In choosing partnership over control, we can better connect in these challenging moments.

There is a strong link between controlling our children and being controlled by our outer-world systems. Consider that we were all raised within a system we have been plugged into from an early age. I'm talking about a system of rules, laws, hierarchy, power, and authority. These outer-world systems have distinct agendas, but the common thread in each of these agendas is simply to survive by maintaining its authority. In most of these systems, such as school, civic culture, society, etc., we weren't asked permission to participate. This is considered a form of colonization. In fact, most of us were expected to go to school, get a job, pay taxes, get married, buy property, and follow a plan laid out by our culture. For most of us, we never were asked to opt in; we were just absorbed into the system based on expectation.

Understanding the nature of the world is a huge task, but bringing in conversations about sovereignty, autonomy, and consent will help us and our teens to navigate these issues with greater awareness. This is part of the conditioning we must claim sovereignty over and decolonize within our own minds.

Seeking Other Support

There are times when we recognize we just can't do this alone. I urge you to seek support if you feel overwhelmed or unsure how to proceed. There is absolutely no shame in it. I've prepared a robust Suggested Reading section at the back of this book, which covers many different topics if you want to learn more. Consider finding a mentor for your teen or enroll them in a course that teaches tools like the ones in this book. Check out my courses and mentorship offerings at Transformative Mentoring for Teens https://transformativementoringforteens.com. If you feel like you need more help, therapy is a wonderful option. When looking for a therapist, please consider seeking someone who is familiar with either of these two methodologies: Cognitive Behavioral Therapy or Acceptance and Commitment Therapy.

Cognitive Behavioral Therapy

Cognitive Behavioral Therapy (CBT) came into prominence over the last forty years as an effective therapeutic approach for greater mental health. Research and validation have shown CBT to be effective with various problems including mood disorders, anxiety, depression, as well as personality and behavioral disorders. Like much of the work I do, CBT focuses on our pattern of thoughts, which stem from our experiences and perceptions. Our thoughts often create belief systems about ourselves, our abilities, and our self-worth translated through our behaviors, fears, anxiety, depression, dependence, or disassociation.

Unlike other traditional therapies, CBT has been the subject of more than 400 clinical trials involving a broad range of conditions, populations, and age groups. CBT has been shown to be as useful as antidepressant medication for individuals with depression and appears to be superior to medication in preventing relapses.

Much of why I like CBT is that it places the responsibility of healing in the hands of the client through tested processes and tools, focusing on the present rather than the past. Although I'm not trained in Cognitive Behavioral Therapy, I have read many books on the topic and have listed a few, including some self-directed CBT workbooks, in the Suggested Reading section.

Like the tools I provide for you in this book, CBT requires the client to learn specific skills that can be used to solve problems they are confronted with. It can also help develop skills such as tracking their triggers and set, measure, and achieve legitimate goals. In essence, CBT teaches the client to focus on developing skills to recognize distorted, unrealistic, or limiting thinking, then provides steps and strategies to change that thinking to modify or eliminate the problematic behavior.

The problem with CBT is that its success is based on a customized program designed for each client, usually lasting twenty weeks or longer. Clients need to fully buy into the experience and want to change, as there are tons of assignment-based processing, accountability, experiments, and recording required. A willingness to change is necessary for CBT to be effective and may not be something you can casually facilitate with your teen. However, many of the tools I've designed for my courses and share in this book are based on the principles of CBT.

Here are the principles of CBT I find valuable. Please keep these ideas in mind as you start to work with the tools in this book, both for yourself and eventually as the facilitator of your teen.

Here are three principles of CBT I find most important:

- Psychological problems are based, in part, on faulty or unhelpful ways of thinking.
- Psychological problems are based, in part, on learned patterns of unhelpful behavior.
- People suffering from psychological problems can learn better ways of coping with them, thereby relieving their symptoms and becoming more effective in their lives.

CBT usually involves efforts to change thinking patterns. These strategies may include:

- Learning to recognize one's distortions in thinking that are creating problems, and then reevaluate them in light of reality.
- Gaining a better understanding of the behavior and motivation of others.
- Using problem-solving skills to cope with difficult situations.
- Learning to develop a greater sense of confidence in one's own abilities.

CBT usually involves efforts to change behavioral patterns. These strategies may include:

- Facing one's fears instead of avoiding them.
- Using role-playing to prepare for potentially problematic interactions with others.
- Learning to calm one's mind and relax one's body.

Acceptance and Commitment Therapy

Acceptance and Commitment Therapy (ACT) is also an action-oriented approach that stems from both traditional behavior therapy and CBT. Much like CBT, clients must face their inner emotions and stop avoiding, denying, and struggling with them. The acceptance part of ACT is learning that the deeper feelings they are experiencing are appropriate responses to their life situations, which helps us deal with judgment and shame. With acceptance as the underlying quality of ACT, clients are supported to accept their hardships and commit to making necessary changes in their behavior, regardless of how they feel about it.

Working with an ACT therapist, clients learn to listen to their own self-talk. If you or your teen has a loud inner voice, this type of therapy is especially effective. Through learning to listen without judgment to the way you talk to yourself, especially surrounding past traumas, problematic relationships, limitations in life situations, or other issues, you can better determine if an issue requires immediate action or must be accepted for what it is.

Behavioral changes are also part of the foundation of ACT. Most clients work with a therapist to design strategies to stop repeating thought patterns and behaviors that cause stress in one's life. Through acceptance, clients learn to make a commitment to stop fighting the past and start practicing more confident and positive behaviors, based on their personal values and goals, in the present.

The reason I like ACT so much is because this style of therapy looks directly at our painful emotions and psychological experiences, and instead of trying to control them, it focuses on accepting and integrating them into our perception of self. Much like we explored through shadow work, our shameful emotions or disowned parts of self never disappear. ACT helps to bring these parts of ourselves into the light through radical acceptance. Once these parts are accepted, we can start integrating our emotional wounds and taking steps to change our behavior.

Final Tools

Congratulations! Give yourself a high five for getting to the end of the book! I know this took tremendous commitment, and I'm certain you found yourself triggered or uneasy with some of its content. Thank you for allowing me to be a part of your journey in supporting greater mental health in your family. I hope this book provided a guide to empower your teen to truly be seen, heard, and understood for the amazing person they are. I support your commitment to building a new, stronger connection with your teen.

Now, the real work begins.

Here is a list of my final nine tools designed to get you started implementing right now. Be patient with yourself and commit to the process. *You got this.*

1. **Listen:** Really, listen to your teen. What does it mean to hold space? Be aware of your triggers, make sure you are really seeing, hearing, and understanding your teen without an agenda or judgment.
   Exercise suggestion: Notice triggers, then inhale deeply, followed by a deep exhale. Take three breaths before responding to regulate your lymphatic system. Make pausing a part of your daily practice.

2. **Choose connection over coercion:** Put your ego aside and don't push to be right or insist on having your way. Ask yourself, does what I'm about to say promote connection, or is it meant to coerce them?
   Exercise suggestion: Set an alarm notification titled, "Would you like to chat/talk?" on your phone. Then, ask your teen this question at the same time, each and every day. Accept "no" as a perfectly acceptable answer. If you are lucky to receive a "yes" answer, sit without an agenda and ask open-ended questions like:
   "What's going on in your life now?"
   "What's alive for you now?"
   "How are you feeling?"

3. **Assess your current opinion about your teen/tween:** Notice where this feeling comes from. Hint: it's normally a situation where you create a judgment about their character. Although the thing that happened may have been true, the opinion you have about them does not allow them to become anything else. If you treat them as someone

who steals or lies because they once did that three years ago, you're not allowing them to realign or reinvent themselves.

> *Exercise suggestion:* Exhale, then get honest. What story do you tell yourself about your teen? Journal it. Examine it. Realize how these opinions are affecting your relationship. Remember this moment and access it again in your mind in real-time when you fall back to these old belief patterns. Are you finding it difficult to forgive and forget? Why?

4. **Help your teen/tween lead more in their lives:** Give them space to empower themselves and be independent. Discuss this with them. Allow space for them to fail, succeed, and quit as they see fit.

> *Exercise suggestion:* Let your teen/tween know this is your intention and ask them how they wish to lead more. Listen to their suggestions and notice how uncomfortable that makes you (that's your work). Engage in dialogue about support, expectations, and consequences. Partner with them to empower them.

5. **Lighten up:** Laugh; bring playfulness into your home, relationship, and family.

> *Exercise suggestion:* Explore what brings playfulness into your family. Really investigate what that is, what that looks like, and what it involves. Do a survey with every member of your family when you are all together, maybe over a meal. Then, challenge everyone to show up for a scheduled time to have fun! Rinse and repeat.

6. **Be the person your teen wants to talk to:** If you are always being critical or judgmental or if all your interactions have an agenda attached, they will never open up with you. You should be viewed as a kind and compassionate person.

> *Exercise suggestion:* One of the principles of connection is to show yourself for who you really are. Share the journey you took to get here. Don't be afraid of sharing your own shortcomings and accessing your place of vulnerability.

7. **Don't solve your teen's problems:** Contrary to popular belief, your teens don't want you to solve their problems. As parents, we often default to being the problem solver because we don't want our teens to struggle. However, by solving their problems, we are robbing them of the experience of critical thinking, decision-making, and learning to listen to their own inner-guidance system. Finally, if we solve their problems for them, we are preventing them from failing in a safe space, an experience everyone must have in order to grow.

   Exercise suggestion: When your teen is faced with a problem, ask them this question, "How can I support you?" From personal experience, I can tell you this question frustrated my son, but it made him accountable for speaking his truth and sharing his own needs. The hardest thing you'll experience as a parent of an adolescent is actually letting them fail.

8. **Don't see your teen as who they were; see them as who they are now:** Don't hold the past against them. What this really means is, as parents, we can't help but see our children as a cumulative experience. We know they were a baby, we know they maybe had rough periods of behavior, etc., but we subconsciously label them as all of these experiences and faults. At this moment, they may have already outgrown all these things. By holding onto those past ideas, we hold them back from being who they are in this moment.

   Exercise suggestion: Recognize you have a normal bias and correct it or just let it go so they can be free to try on new identities. Remember, this is a time of tremendous development and change. Because they are the ones who once did _____ (fill in the blank), your current beliefs about them are biased. Drop it. Look at them as a new human who was born on this day with a completely clean slate.

9. **Rewrite your family's story:** Stories play a tremendous role in the family dynamic, requiring participants to become comfortable being open and honest about their own stories. Know your story and do your own healing for your teen to know their story and do their healing.

Exercise suggestion: With your teen, co-create your family story, which doesn't have to be based on the reality of what is currently happening at this very moment. The story can be based on your aspirations or desires. What do I mean by this? Together figure out the answer to this statement:
"We are a family who _____."
It can be the new story of how you interact, how you feel, and how you take on the world together.

Parents, I am inviting you to share your experiences reading *Seen, Heard & Understood: Parenting & Partnering with Teens for Greater Mental Health* with me.

I'd love to know how this book supported greater connection in your family. Please share how it felt to step into partnership with your adolescent and the ways your families transformed. How did the tools work for you?

Please send your messages, testimonials and stories to book@transformativementoringforteens.com

I can't wait to connect with you!

Sincerely yours, in partnership,

Lainie Liberti

Acknowledgments

I wish to acknowledge the following people who contributed one way or another to the making of this book. Without you, none of this would have been possible.

Miro Siegel: You are the reason this book was written. You have inspired me every single day to be a better person, heal my wounds, and to be radically accountable. Thank you for choosing me to be your mom.

Greg Gronowski: Thank you for trusting me and my intuition. Thank you for knowing it was okay to raise our son on a different path. Thank you for granting us this adventure. You are so deeply missed.

Quinn McKinney: Your creative spirit and commitment to doing the inner work inspires me daily, and I'm so blessed to have you as my mentee and assistant in this work. Keep writing and keep trusting yourself. It's been such an honor to watch your transition into adulthood. I see you. I hear you. I understand you.

Gianna Cino: I've had the pleasure of meeting you at 18 on your first trip out of the US. I'm so grateful you decided to trust me, travel, and volunteer with me over a five-year period, exploring Peru, Greece, Thailand, Japan, and Mexico together. I'm privileged to have witnessed your transformation into the beautiful adult you have become, and it's an honor to call you a friend.

Matthew Harms: Thank you for being the best writing coach and believing in this book. Thank you for putting up with me most Fridays, pushing me when I was stuck (constantly) and giving me deadlines (which I always missed). Without your support, all of this would still be a dream.

Marissa Blose: Thank you for your editing genius, bringing your own passion for these topics, and your amazing insights.

Estrella Labrada: Deepest gratitude for the beautiful cover art and illustrations found within this book. Your talent helped to tell a story to all the parents who have committed to supporting their teens.

Dr. Zoltan Nadasdy: Thank you for the intro into the brain and for making the subject so accessible to me for years to come. You'll never know the impact you've had on my life.

Sarah Beale: Fellow anarchist, thank you for partnering with me to support so many parents starting in 2020. Thank you for sharing with me your heart, your spirit, your experiences, and your cherished friendship. Through our conversations, you helped breathe partnership parenting into reality and how to describe it from our many hours and hours of laughter-filled Zoom conversations. I love you, and I'm hoping we'll get the chance to have that gin and tonic in person together very soon.

Robin Engstrom: Thank you for more than 50 years of friendship, including our numerous teen adventures, finding all kinds of trouble, cruising around in your purple Pacer, and always rocking out to Oingo Boingo. Thank you most of all for our heartfelt conversations as I was writing this book, confirming my most difficult memories from childhood and reminding me that we both did the best we could possibly do.

Lauren Siegel: I want to express my deepest gratitude for my Pops. I love being your daughter. I'm happy we found each other again in my adulthood, and I'm grateful for your support, bad jokes, and your twisted sense of humor. Most of all, I'm beyond thrilled you finally found the love of your life, Edi, and are living in partnership with a woman who brings out the best in you!

I especially want to acknowledge all of the teens past, present, and future, who I have had the honor of working with. All of you have touched my life in the most profound way and have given meaning to my life. It hasn't always been easy or comfortable, but thank you for letting me in, allowing me to see you, hear you, and understand you all. I truly love you all:

Abi, Abigail, Adam, Adlai, Aidan, Aidan T., Akilah, Alan, Alex, Aloys, Amalie, Aradan, Aria O., Aria P., Ash R., Ash S., Ashley,

Ashton, Aura, Austin, Avery, Azalia, Azra, Benjamin, Ben, Betty Lou, Blue, Bode, Brahm, Brandon, Cadie, Camden, Cami, Carter, Cassidy, Claire, Clare, Colton, Crew, Daniel, Dani, Danni, David, Dereje, Dominic, Dustin, Dylan, Echo, Eliot, Enver, Erin, Essa, Esther, Ethan, Eva, Evan, Ezra, Faith, Gabriella, Genna, Georgina, Gianna, Gil, Griffin, Haven, Haley, Harrison N., Harrison T., Howard, Hudson, Imani, Isadora, J, Jacob C, Jacob K., Jaci, Jack, Jaden F., Jaden M., Jake, Jarod, Jasmine, Jasper, Javen, Jerick, Jess, Jonah, Josh, June, Justyna, Juwayria, Kaitlin, Kaitlyn, Kamil, Katie J., Katie M., Katie McD., Kaya, Kaylin, Kegan, Keira, Kemaya, Kerry, Kiai, Kieran, Kira, Korbin, Kurt, Leilani, Liam, Logan D., Logan S., Lorien, Lucy, Lyra, Madeleine, Madison, Mae, Mateo, Matthew C., Matthew M., Maya, Miah, Mida, Moo, Nagumi, Noah, Nova, Oliver B., Oliver K., Paola, Phoenix, Quin, Rainer, Red, Reece, Reid, Remme, Riley, Rio, Ryan, Rylei, Sadie, Samone, Sam L., Sam W., Salem, Sarah, Shanee, Shane, Sienna, Skelly, Slater, Sydney, Tamir, Tcherari, Tesh, Thomas D., Thomas J., Tito, Toast, Toby, Tomacz, Tuilerie, Veer, Victoria, Vlad, Wednesday, Wiley, William, Vlad, Xanthe

Finally, to my Mother, thank you. You've given me the gift of healing. I love you.

Suggested Reading

I am honored to provide you with a robust reading list to support your continued journey inward. We are always healing, growing, and transforming. I've read or listened to most of the books on this list, and for the ones I have not, they came highly recommended to me, and I will eventually get to them. Please enjoy.

Anxiety, Depression & Stress

Feeling Great: The Revolutionary New Treatment for Depression and Anxiety
By David D. Burns MD

Feeling Good: The New Mood Therapy
By David D. Burns MD

The End of Mental Illness: How Neuroscience Is Transforming Psychiatry and Helping Prevent or Reverse Mood and Anxiety Disorders, ADHD, Addictions, PTSD, Psychosis, Personality Disorders, and More
By Daniel G. Amen

When the Body Says No: The Cost of Hidden Stress
By Gabor Maté

The Stress Switch: The Truth About Stress and How to Short-Circuit It
By Dr. Amy Serin

Attachment Theory

This suggested reading list is provided courtesy of Dr. Kate Green, attachment specialist https://drkategreen.com

The Attachment Parenting Book: A Commonsense Guide to Understanding and Nurturing Your Baby
By William Sears, Martha Sears

Why Love Matters: How Affection Shapes a Baby's Brain
By Sue Gerhardt

The Neuroscience of Human Relationships: Attachment And the Developing Social Brain
By Louis Cozolino

The Developing Mind: How Relationships and the Brain Interact to Shape Who We Are
By Daniel J. Siegel

Strange Situation: A Mother's Journey Into the Science of Attachment
By Bethany Saltman

Handbook of Attachment: Theory, Research, and Clinical Applications
By Jude Cassidy

Attachment-Focused Parenting: Effective Strategies to Care for Children
By Daniel A. Hughes

Our Babies Ourselves
By Meredith Small

Maternal-Infant Bonding
By John Kennell Marshall Klaus

Becoming Attached: First Relationships and How They Shape Our Capacity to Love
> By Robert Karen

Attachment Parenting: Instinctive Care for Your Baby and Young Child
> By Katie Allison Granju, Betsy Kennedy, William Sears

A Secure Base
> By John Bowlby

Infancy In Uganda, Infant Care and the Growth of Love
> By Mary Ainsworth

Patterns of Attachment: A Psychological Study of the Strange Situation (Psychology Press & Routledge Classic Editions) 1st Edition
> By Mary D. Salter Ainsworth, Mary C. Blehar, Everett Waters, Sally N. Wall

CBT

The CBT Workbook for Mental Health: Evidence-Based Exercises to Transform Negative Thoughts and Manage Your Well-Being
> By Simon Rego PsyD, Sarah Fader

Retrain Your Brain: Cognitive Behavioral Therapy in 7 Weeks: A Workbook for Managing Depression and Anxiety
> By Seth J. Gillihan

Anxiety Relief for Teens: Essential CBT Skills and Mindfulness Practices to Overcome Anxiety and Stress
> By Regine Galanti PhD

Childism

Childism: Confronting Prejudice Against Children
By Elizebeth Young-Breuhl

Conflict Resolution

Nonviolent Communication: Create Your Life, Your Relationships, and Your World in Harmony with Your Values
By Marshall Rosenberg PhD

Nonviolent Communication: A Language of Life: Life-Changing Tools for Healthy Relationships (Nonviolent Communication Guides)
By Marshall Rosenberg PhD

Journaling Books for Teens

Goodbye, Anxiety: A Guided Journal for Overcoming Worry (A Guided Workbook for Teens and Young Adults with CBT Skills and Journal Prompts)
By Terri Bacow Ph.D.

Teen Journaling: Top Ten: Over 100 Prompts to Spark Creative Journal Pages (Journaling Prompts Book 1)
By April Sanes

Wreck This Journal: Now in Color
By Keri Smith

Let That Sh*t Go: A Journal for Leaving Your Bullsh*t Behind and Creating a Happy Life (Zen as F*ck Journals)
By Monica Sweeney

The No Worries Workbook: 124 Lists, Activities, and Prompts to Get Out of Your Head—and On with Your Life! Paperback
By Molly Burford

Mindfulness

Growing Up Mindful: Essential Practices to Help Children, Teens, and Families Find Balance, Calm, and Resilience
By Christopher Willard

Parenting

The Conscious Parent: Transforming Ourselves, Empowering Our Children
By Dr. Shefali Tsabary

Unconditional Parenting: Moving from Rewards and Punishments to Love and Reason
By Alfie Kohn

Raising Human Beings
By Ross W. Greene

The Explosive Child
By Ross W. Greene

Hold On to Your Kids: Why Parents Need to Matter More Than Peers
By Gordon Neufeld & Gabor Mate

Parenting from the Inside Out: How a Deeper Self-Understanding Can Help You Raise Children Who Thrive
By Daniel J. Siegel , Mary Hartzell

The Power of Showing Up: How Parental Presence Shapes Who Our Kids Become and How Their Brains Get Wired
By Daniel J. Siegel MD, Tina Payne Bryson PhD

The Conscious Parent: Transforming Ourselves, Empowering Our Children
By Dr. Shefali Tsabar

The Continuum Concept: In Search of Happiness Lost (Classics in Human Development)
    By Jean Liedloff

Parenting for a Peaceful World
    By Robin Grille

Raising Our Children, Raising Ourselves: Transforming Parent-Child Relationship from Reaction and Struggle to Freedom, Power and Joy
    By Naomi Aldort

The Gifts of Imperfect Parenting: Raising Children with Courage, Compassion, and Connection
    By Brené Brown

Consciously Parenting: What it Really Takes to Raise Emotionally Healthy Families
    By Rebecca Thompson M.S.

Creating Connection: Essential Tools for Growing Families through Conception, Birth and Beyond (Consciously Parenting Book 2)
    By Rebecca Thompson

Nurturing Connection: What Parents Need to Know About Emotional Expression and Bonding (Consciously Parenting Book 3)
    By Rebecca Thompson

Peaceful Parent, Happy Kids
    By Dr. Laura Markham

Kids Are Worth It!: Giving Your Child the Gift of Inner Discipline
    By Barbara Coloroso

Self-Healing & Tools

The Emotionally Absent Mother: How to Recognize and Heal the Invisible Effects of Childhood Emotional Neglect, Second Edition
By Jasmin Lee Cori MS LPC

The Road Back to Me: Healing and Recovering from Co-Dependency, Addiction, Enabling, and Low Self Esteem
By Lisa A. Romano

How to Do the Work: Recognize Your Patterns, Heal from Your Past, and Create Your Self
By Dr. Nicole LePera

Are u ok?: A Guide to Caring for Your Mental Health
By Kati Morton, LMFT

How to Develop Your Self-Confidence: Effective Help Guide to Create and Grow Self-Esteem: The Healing Power of Love, Empathy, and Compassion
By Brian James

Loving What Is: Four Questions That Can Change Your Life
By Byron Katie

The Power of Now
By Eckhart Tolle

The High 5 Habit: Take Control of Your Life with One Simple Habit
By Mel Robbins

The 5 Second Rule: Transform your Life, Work, and Confidence with Everyday Courage
By Mel Robbins

The Biology of Belief: Unleashing the Power of Consciousness, Matter & Miracles

By Bruce H. Lipton

Becoming Supernatural: How Common People Are Doing the Uncommon
By Joe Dispenza

SuperWellness: Become Your Own Best Healer; The Revolutionary New Formula for Creating True Vibrant Health
By Dr. Edith Ubuntu Chan

Shadows

The Dark Side of the Light Chasers
By Debbie Ford

The Secret of the Shadow: The Power of Owning Your Whole Story
By Debbie Ford

The Shadow Effect: Illuminating the Hidden Power of Your True Self
By Debbie Ford, Deepak Chopra, and Marianne Williamson

SHADOW WORK JOURNAL FOR BEGINNERS: Shadow Work Prompts Journal and Workbook for Beginners
By Meadow Belle

Shame

I Thought It Was Just Me (but it isn't): Telling the Truth about Perfectionism, Inadequacy, and Power
By Brené Brown

Braving the Wilderness: The Quest for True Belonging and the Courage to Stand Alone
By Brené Brown

The Gifts of Imperfection
By Brené Brown

Teens

Brainstorm: The Power and the Purpose of Teenage Brain
By Daniel Siegel

The Teenage Liberation Handbook: How to Quit School and Get a Real Life and Education
By Grace Llewellyn

Available Parent: Expert Advice for Raising Successful and Resilient Teens and Tweens
By Dr. Duffy John

How to Hug a Porcupine: Negotiating the Prickly Points of the Tween Years
By Julie A. Ross

The Grown-Up's Guide to Teenage Humans: How to Decode Their Behavior, Develop Trust, and Raise a Respectable Adult
By Josh Shipp

TEENS Unleashed: Unschooling Young Adults as They Reach for Their Dreams
By Karla Williams

Trauma

What Happened to You?: Conversations on Trauma, Resilience, and Healing
By Oprah Winfrey & Bruce D. Perry

Worthy: A Personal Guide for Healing Your Childhood Trauma
By Josephine Faulk MPH

The Body Keeps the Score: Brain, Mind, and Body in the Healing of Trauma
By Bessel van der Kolk

It Didn't Start with You: How Inherited Family Trauma Shapes Who We Are and How to End the Cycle
By Mark Wolynn

Unschooling

Free to Learn
By Peter Gray

Unschooled: Raising Curious, Well-Educated Children Outside the Conventional Classroom
By Kerry McDonald

Unschooling: Exploring Learning Beyond the Classroom (Palgrave Studies in Alternative Education)
By Gina Riley

Teach Your Own: The Indispensable Guide to Living and Learning with Children at Home
By John Holt and Pat Farenga

How Children Learn, 50th Anniversary Edition
By John Holt

How Children Fail
By John Holt

Passion-Driven Education: How to Use Your Child's Interests to Ignite a Lifelong Love of Learning
By Connor Boyack

Raising Free People: Unschooling as Liberation and Healing Work
By Akilah S. Richards and Bayo Akomolafe

The Unschooling Journey: A Field Guide
By Pam Laricchia

Homeschooled Teens: 75 Young People Speak About Their Lives Without School
By Sue Patterson

Why Are You Still Sending Your Kids to School?
By Blake Boles

About the Author

Lainie is an author, speaker, community leader, teen coach, and alternative education advocate who helped to spearhead the thriving worldschooling movement.

After the 2008 California economy crash, Liberti closed her Los Angeles-based branding agency. Liberti and her then 9-year-old son Miro decided to be the change instead of the victims by choosing a life of adventure. After selling all of their possessions, Liberti and her son hit the road for what was meant to be a one-year adventure. Thirteen years and almost 50 countries later, the pair has since settled in Mexico. Lainie chose to educate her son Miro through the world by facilitating rich experiential learning, cultural immersion, volunteering, and leadership as his school. The pair are often credited with birthing what's known as the modern worldschooling movement. Over the years, Liberti has worked tirelessly as an advocate to bring worldschooling into public awareness and become part of the alternative education conversation.

Liberti has spoken about worldschooling on the TEDxEdu stage in Amsterdam, has written about learning through travel for multiple magazines, academic journals, and websites including *International Journal of Education, Journal of Unschooling and Alternative Learning, People Magazine, Huffington Post, USA Today, The New York Times,* and *The New York Post,* and has contributed to several books on the topic of worldschooling.

Lainie cofounded Project World School with her son in 2012. Liberti designs and co-facilitates the Project World School teen retreats as month-long immersive learning communities to support self-directed teens from around the world. Over the years, Lainie has facilitated more than 20 international retreats for almost 100 teens, learning through cultural immersion, examining personal values, and exploring world views.

Lainie Liberti is also the founder and creator of Transformative Mentoring for Teens that launched in early 2020, offering virtual 1:1 coaching for teens as well as a 12-week course designed to transform lives. Lainie is a certified life coach, specializing in transformational coaching.

In addition, Lainie founded Project World School Family Summits, where she has produced nine in-person international conferences for hundreds of worldschooling families across Europe, Asia, and Mexico since 2016. Lainie also launched the We Are Worldschooling Community Club serving her Facebook community of 11k members and the Virtual Worldschooling Summit in early 2020.

Lainie lives in Mexico with her dog Carlos, enjoys rooftop gardening, and the weekly visits from her son Miro who comes over to do his laundry.

Testimonials:
What Teens and Parents Say

I want to share a few of the testimonials from both parents and teens I've worked with. Their words are more powerful than any words I could write here. For more testimonials, please visit my website at https://transformativementoringforteens.com/

"Lainie is always there. She always has something to offer me no matter what I am going through and that has been so, so lovely." Quinlan Willow, Teen

"I'm so glad to have worked with Lanie NOW. I think everyone needs this now. I wouldn't give it up for the world." - Camilla Downs, Parent

"Lanie is so intuitive in seeing and treating teens at an equal level and does not talk down to them, which is so different from my experience with traditional educators." - Parent

"Lanie has a gift for understanding teens and tweens on an emotional level and tap into their gifts." - Belinda Bonham Carter, Parent

"The tools Lanie used with my children are hard to find in mainstream society and we refer back to them all the time to bring new concepts into our family." - Belinda Bonham Carter. Parent

"Lanie really has a special gift for honoring all children equally and bringing them together no matter their differences." - Alexandra Rosela, Parent

"I didn't know my daughter was suicidal until after a few months of working with Lanie when she was comfortable enough to tell me." - Taryn Helper, Parent

"The individual work helped my daughter know herself better and understand everyone her age is going through the same changes. It reinforced that everything was going to be ok and increased her confidence." - Sandra Vincent, Parent

"The best part of mentoring was being able to get deeper into myself and learn more about my feelings, interests, and learn more on how to identify what I was feeling." - Teen

"I cannot say enough wonderful things about this course!! My eldest daughter is just finishing the 12-week course and has enjoyed every minute of it, and looked forward to the weekly sessions. I've watched her reignite her excitement for new projects and really expand her confidence levels. I highly recommend this course to parents who have worldschooling teens. Lainie's ability to really connect with the young people and to guide them to deeper personal discovery is amazing and priceless."
-Dani A., Parent

"I learned I don't have to agree with others, it's ok to disagree." - Teen

"There was so much to learn from the experiences of others my age and some I never would have thought to reach out to on my own." - Teen

Notes

Please use this space to write notes as you read this book.

Lainie Liberti

Made in United States
Troutdale, OR
07/04/2023

10963843R00184